Women and Loss

The Foundation of Thanatology Series, Volume 3

Other Volumes in the Series

Women and Loss

Psychobiological Perspectives

edited by

William F. Finn
Margot Tallmer
Irene B. Seeland
Austin H. Kutscher

and

Elizabeth J. Clark

With the Assistance of
Lillian Kutscher

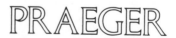

PRAEGER SPECIAL STUDIES • PRAEGER SCIENTIFIC

New York • Philadelphia • Eastbourne, UK
Toronto • Hong Kong • Tokyo • Sydney

Library of Congress Cataloging in Publication Data

Main entry under title:
Women and loss.

(The Foundation of Thanatology series ; v. 3)
Includes bibliographies and index.
1. Gynecology—Psychological aspects.   2. Women—
Psychology.   3. Deprivation (Psychology)   4. Bereavement.
5. Death—Psychological aspects.   I. Finn, William F.
II. Kutscher, Lillian G.   III. Series: Foundation of
Thanatology series (Praeger Publishers) ; v. 3.
RG103.5.W66   1985   155.9′16   84-23725
ISBN 0-03-070646-7 (alk. paper)

WMN
RG 103.5
W66
1985

Published in 1985 by Praeger Publishers
CBS Educational and Professional Publishing
a Division of CBS Inc.
521 Fifth Avenue, New York, NY 10175 USA
© 1985 by Praeger Publishers

56789 052 987654321

Printed in the United States of America
on acid-free paper

Thanatology is a discipline whose focus is on the practice of supportive physical and emotional care for those who are life-threatened, with an equal concern exhibited for the well-being of their family members. Proposed is a philosophy of care giving that reinforces alternative ways of enhancing the quality of life, that introduces methods of intervention on behalf of the emotional status of all involved, that fosters a more mature understanding of the dying process and the problems of separation, loss, bereavement, and grief.

The editors wish to acknowledge the support and encouragement of the Foundation of Thanatology in the preparation of this book. All royalties from its sale are directly assigned to this not-for-profit, tax exempt, public, scientific, and educational foundation.

Preface

Normal biological processes, unpredictable physical pathologies, and psychological stresses all create problems that may require professional intervention. Of particular relevance in women's lives are the physical changes subsumed under the category "gynecologic complications," the psychosocial changes accompanying the individual woman's role as a daughter, wife, mother, widow, or participant in a professional milieu. Psychological stresses emanate from both of these or are responsible in part for them.

This book presents overviews from psychobiological perspectives as a means of calling attention to situations that require the most sensitive of supportive care giving from the most knowledgeable of care givers. Thus, by anticipating the problems that alter an individual's functioning, informed care givers can provide prophylactic efforts, therapeutic care, and preventive intervention to ease the impact of unfortunate circumstances when they intrude into the lives of women.

It is not our intention to provide a litany of traumatic and tragic events. Rather, the purpose of this book is to arouse consciousness about the negative potential of certain events on the woman (and, as a consequence, on her family and community) and to suggest guidelines for the kind of compassionate care that is every person's entitlement.

With or without equal rights in the home, marketplace, or political arena, women are the source of stability for most families. The dynamics of the physical and emotional functioning of the woman imposes a structure within the household that affects spouse and children. Even though women in greater numbers have become "liberated" from specific and traditional home-oriented tasks, nothing can change their role as child bearers or alter the mortality statistics that mark them as widowed survivors. Life encompasses multiple situations where choice is not a factor, where sex is the determinant of status and function.

Contributing to this book are multidisciplinary care givers who, through professional training and life experiences, have developed expertise for diagnosing the ills of the body and the spirit, for reversing in as many ways as possible the destructiveness of these ills, for preventing their occurrence, and for rehabilitation when the best of preventive measures and therapeutic care falls short of restoring "wellness." Although it is usually most difficult or impossible to transform certain losses into gains, a realistic approach to many of these losses can invest life with positive dimensions that reinforce relationships, foster growth, and enhance the quality of daily living for everyone.

Contents

PART II

MISCARRIAGE, PERINATAL DEATH,

AND ABORTION

PART III

LIFE-THREATENING ILLNESS

AND BODY IMAGE

Part I
The Facts of Life
for Women

1

The Normal Losses
of Being Female

Lila J. Kalinich

The whole of feminine psychology can be organized around the theme of loss. Even traditional Freudian concepts, which many feminists today dispute, seem to contain this rather poignant intuition about the nature of a woman's life. Little girls, said Freud, believe that they once had something—a penis—that they were forced to give up. "Is Mother responsible?" they ask. Freud called this self-assessment feelings of castration and, as a result, he described penis envy. He meant these terms both concretely and symbolically, in effect stating that a perceived (misperceived) loss dictated the formation of the feminine psyche.

However, by the time a little girl's consciousness is sufficiently developed to even ponder issues of loss and difference, she is already aware that in order to stay the course of healthy maturation as a female, she must relinquish her mother as the object of her passion and turn to her father. Although this shift in love object is accompanied by a measure of relief from the pressures of psychological closeness, it is concurrently experienced as a loss. The mother of those early years is retrieved only much later in life, through the process of mothering itself.

This loss is only the first of many uniquely feminine ones that the woman experiences throughout her life.

When one talks about women as a group, one runs the risk of being accused of misunderstanding men. To talk about women and loss does not imply that loss is an insignificant factor in the lives of men. Men have their losses, potential and real, too. But perhaps the timing and the content of the issues are somewhat different.

To consider things in a very simple way, we can create a hypothetical little girl and walk her through life. We have already taken her through the early years when she has discovered that she must give up her passionate and sexual attachment to her mother if she is to become an ordinary woman. As she approaches three to six years of age, she intensifies her attachment to her father and he becomes her love object. She develops the so-called Oedipus or Electra complex. But again, the requirements of reality intervene, and she comes to understand that an actual conscious sexual attitude is not permissible by ordinary standards. And again she confronts a loss.

Freud claimed that women never truly relinquish this tie to father. He formulated this, too, in terms of a penis metaphor. Boys have something to lose, really: the male genital. Girls do not. The male's fear that, in fact, he might be castrated if he does not yield in the competition with father for mother, enforces the resolution of the Oedipus complex. Girls, Freud said, have nothing to lose. Hence, they are less intimidated by reality; their Oedipus resolution remains incomplete. Although it does seem correct that women do hold onto their fathers, sometimes for dear life, Freud's explanation of this phenomenon is at best partial, despite its grain of truth.

The hypothetical little girl then enters what is usually called the latency period. According to classical thinking, latency—which begins approximately age six—is a time when infantile instinctual drives go into remission. Its years are usually marked by quiet, industrious activity when new skills are acquired and real strengths in managing them are developed. For instance, most children begin to read at this time. In a sense, latency represents childhood at its best. For most children it is a happy, rewarding time. However, for our little girl it can be relatively short-lived. She will soon face the abrupt end of the relatively trouble-free time, in effect facing the loss of her childhood with the onset of menarche.

The menstrual period seems to be appearing in progressively younger girls these days. It is not uncommon to find ten-, nine-, and even eight-year-olds who are menstruating. With menarche, the epiphyses, or growth centers of the bones, close, so that for the most part the girl no longer grows in height. Contrast this with the male, for whom puberty arrives more gradually and heralds a growth spurt. For the girl, something is clearly and definitively over as she arrives at early adulthood. Usually, the excited anticipation of what is to come in her life serves as the overriding feeling that accompanies menarche and puberty, but the loss of childhood must be integrated as well. Many women later recall feeling that this was the beginning of the end.

As our little girl enters adolescence, she probably will benefit from a moratorium. Despite the potential for problems with school, conflicts with parents, and the emotional hazards of encountering sexuality, most adolescents are fairly happy and involved in exploring themselves and the world. Our little girl in all likelihood will taste bits of, and certainly dream of, the sugarplums that life has to offer. She will set out to plan the perfect life: a most rewarding career, a most glorious romance, a most satisfying marriage, the most beautiful children, a most fulfilling vocational achievement, and great public recognition.

However, she will once again confront the impositions of reality. First, as she embarks on her sexual life, she will lose her virginity. As she selects a spouse, under traditional circumstances she will lose her last name. And almost because of the rich multiplicity of options she has available as a contemporary woman, she will have to make choices that will require her to give up a part of herself. Despite compensating rewards, she will experience this giving-up as a loss.

Should she choose to pursue a career, she will have to decide just how to do it. Will she devote herself to it completely, or will she choose to have a family as well? Should she seek the former, she will inevitably have to come to grips with the loss of the part of her that has been anticipating the possibility of motherhood. Should she go the route of motherhood and family, she will sacrifice some part of her career. If she has children and still pursues her career, she will lose something in her relationship with her children.

If our little girl does marry and have children, she will know soon enough what it means to be swept away by motherly love. Somewhat like the female spider who dies after she lays her eggs, she will allow her own identity to recede as she immerses herself in the care of her young. She will experience a loss of independence and personal significance as well as a loss of her own time. She will become acquainted with deference as her own sense of pleasure and preference becomes less important. The notion of deference implies something more than a voluntary act of self-surrender. Deference is an ego state, a state of being characterized by an involuntary constriction of a part of the personality, a loss of the part that chooses, wishes, hopes, and dreams.

Even as our little girl, now an adult woman, makes the decision to try to become pregnant, she invests her anticipated baby with special feelings. Whether or not she will in fact be fertile becomes an anxiety-producing question. Will she encounter a loss of all that fantasied potential? When she conceives, she must then confront the genuine precariousness of pregnancy. She may miscarry. She may undergo the tragedy of a stillborn baby or a neonatal death. Or she may have a voluntary abortion. In the latter case, the chances are that she will not experience the loss of that terminated pregnancy until she carries a baby whom she wants to keep, but the feelings will be there nevertheless. Perhaps she may have an amniocentesis that reveals genetic abnormalities in the fetus and then decide to terminate the pregnancy. These are very sad circumstances for fathers as well, but most people will agree that as the mother carries the child, so does she also carry the grief.

If we assume that a happy outcome is ensured for our little girl, she has her career, her marriage, and the desired number of wonderful children who live happy, healthy lives. As she enters the years when having additional children becomes unlikely or impossible, she may experience some sadness at the loss of her childbearing capacity. This is especially true, as can be imagined, for the woman who has chosen not to be a mother. At this juncture, she may question her decision. But even with children, the mother may think about those potential young ones who have not come into being. What would additional children have been like? Who would the next child in the bathtub have been?

With menopause comes the loss of the menses. Friend or enemy, it has been a partner, a determiner of much of the rhythm of her life. As its advent symbolized the loss of childhood, its passing symbolizes the anticipation of old age and the end of life. Our little girl is still a middle-aged woman, but she has reached a clear-cut landmark that men often do not experience until they retire. She is definitely over some sort of hill. And her children are probably applying to college, if they are not already there. She will have to confront how much of herself she has given to them. Although the returns may have been plentiful, she may feel somewhat emptied out and spent. She will recall the dreams of her youth and may now keenly experience their loss. If she can give them up in their old form, she will revise them and energize them and find a new sense of freedom. If not, she may undergo a depression.

With all of this behind her, our little girl may still face widowhood. Husbands do tend to die earlier than their wives, showing perhaps that life is harder on men after all. This loss can be overwhelming and disintegrating, especially to the woman who has organized her whole life around husband and family. Even for the woman with a career, this can be true. Furthermore, widows often experience loss of status in the community in the absence of their established husbands.

So there it is: just about one loss in each decade. The experience of, the anticipation of, or the fear of loss seems to provide the counterpoint for a woman's life. And it seems that this manifests itself in a woman's reaction to illness as well. Women tend to become depressed when they are sick.

For example, a common reaction to hysterectomy is a sense of profound loss, even when there is no rational basis such as a desire for additional children. Women describe themselves as feeling empty inside. Obviously, the uterus concretizes something about how they see their lives as women. Some say they fear that their sexual responsiveness will be altered. And sometimes it is—for psychological rather than important physiological reasons.

In contrast, men tend to be more anxious when they are ill—except, of course, when the illness is a catastrophic one. In a way, anxiety is an unconscious effort to avert or prevent a loss, a way of staying vigilant. Women's depression seems to contain an unconscious experience of repeating something old—as if to say, "Oh no, here we go again." It contains a sense of defeat and resignation, feelings that our little girl has had to battle from very early in life.

2

Multiple-Role Women: Issues in Social Negotiations

Barbra Zuck Locker

The number of married women who work has nearly doubled during the past 20 years. Today, 45 percent of married women are employed. An even more salient statistic indicates that 43 percent of employed women have children under the age of six ("The Super-woman Squeeze" (1980). There is every indication that the pattern of combining traditional female roles with careers outside the home will continue (U.S., Department of Commerce 1979). This trend has vastly increased the number of multiple-role women, women who engage in both the traditional wife/mother role and the career role.

The problems that these women face are likely to have widespread implications not only for the women themselves but in relationships between men and women, in the family structure, and in the workplace. It is essential that those in the helping professions have an awareness of the difficult aspects of these problems and how they interface. It certainly appears likely that counseling women and men about coping with changing women's roles will be a major issue in the 1980s (O'Neil 1981; Scarato and Sigall 1979).

The purposes of this chapter are to examine the social changes that have increased women's roles and to explore the effects that involvement in multiple roles has had on women and, to some extent, their families.

CHANGES IN THE SOCIAL STRUCTURE:
ROLE INCREASES FOR WOMEN

Technological advances in contraception, longer life expectancies, the consciousness raising of the women's liberation movement, and the economic recession have all figured prominently in the trend toward multiple roles for women.

Hoffman (1977) saw smaller families and longer lives as contributing to the major shift in a woman's role from essentially that
of a homemaker to a homemaker-worker. Historically, career commitment in the adult life cycle has been made difficult for the female
because of the frequency and unpredictability of pregnancy. Techno-
logically advanced methods of contraception have enabled women to
exercise control over childbearing patterns and family size. In addition, as a result of longer life expectancies, the childbearing and
rearing years occupy less of a woman's life-span than they have in
the past. This leaves many more years for involvement in activities
outside the home. Statistics on the large number of employed mothers
indicate that the time-honored pattern of sequential roles (that is,
career entry or reentry after childbearing is completed) has given
way to simultaneous roles, overlapping career with childbearing.

This transition from single to multiple roles has been largely
influenced by major societal changes brought about by the women's
liberation movement. Since the advent of the women's movement in
the 1960s, there has been growing acceptance of the idea that more
and more women will seek satisfaction from activities unrelated to
marriage and family.

The women's movement has encouraged more options for both
women and men. Through media coverage, consciousness-raising
groups, and a growing feminist literature, the message spread that
it was acceptable to seek fulfillment in a greater expanse of areas.
For women, this has meant a redefinition of the life cycle.

Traditionally, a woman's life cycle has been synonymous with
her family's life cycle. Women have regulated their life course to
the patterns of the family. Marriage and childbearing caused women
to drop out of school or the labor force, and reentry was postponed
until a time in the family's life cycle (when children were grown)
made it possible for them to return. This subservience of the female
life cycle to the family life cycle produced narrow and confining boundaries of stage-appropriate behavior for women. In the past decade
increased knowledge about adult life cycle development has produced
more flexible ideas of stage-appropriate behavior. It is now a more
accepted notion that various activities can be engaged in simultaneously, the family being one of many activities in the life cycle of women
(Hooper 1979). Statistics show an overwhelming increase in the numbers of women participating in higher education and placing a higher
priority on career advancement (Van Dusen and Sheldon 1976).

In addition to (1) the advances in medical technology that have
given women more control over their biology and (2) the socio-cultural-
political influences of the women's movement, an economic factor has
been involved in women's increased participation in the labor force.
The rising cost of living and spiraling inflation have made wives' em-

ployment a necessity for some families. Economic trends mandate the need for the dual-career family in the future.

The combined effect of the major social and economic changes that have influenced the life cycles of women in the United States has enabled them to add involvement in activities outside the family to their traditional roles of wife, mother, and homemaker without sacrificing social acceptance. There are, however, unliberating as well as liberating aspects of multiple roles for the women who engage in them.

DIFFICULTIES OF MULTIPLE-ROLE NEGOTIATION

The social changes that have expanded options for women have also emphasized unique problems. Some areas that warrant exploration are the direct effects that increased roles have on women's lives. Role strain, role conflict, and role overload have been identified as stressful effects of multiple roles on women who have both a career and a family.

ROLE STRAIN, ROLE CONFLICT, AND ROLE OVERLOAD

Role strain has been defined by Goode as the felt difficulty in fulfilling role obligations (1960). It is recognized that all individuals take part in many different role relationships. There are somewhat different responsibilities for each. The individual often contends with conflicting role obligations. It is difficult to perform adequately in one role area if the individual does well in a conflicting role area. Goode concludes that role strain is an inevitable consequence of attempting to meet the demands of the multiplicity of roles that an individual faces.

The conflictual aspects of role strain are clear, but role overload expresses a different dimension of the problem. Role overload describes the acquiring of additional roles beyond the scope of the individual's time and energy limitations. Roles vary in terms of the amount of time and energy needed to fulfill them, and wherever possible, balancing techniques are used to avoid role overloading. The potential for role conflict and/or overload exists for women who combine a career with family obligations. Richardson (1981) recognized that this potential would be greatly influenced by the role context of the role conflict. That is, any discussion of the role conflict brought on by multiple roles must take into consideration the greatly varying circumstances involved in those roles. Richardson contended that the degree of conflict experienced is likely to be influenced both by the structure and organization of the family and by the demands of the occupation engaged in outside the home.

Achievement Patterns and Marriage

Research has indicated that career commitment is stronger among women who are single than among married women (Harmon 1970; Wolfson 1976). One reason for this might be that single women experience less role conflict than married women. Although many factors influence achievement motivation in females (Fitzgerald and Crites 1980), numerous studies have identified role conflict as one of the internal factors hindering occupational aspirations in females, and such conflict has been linked to underachievement and fear of success (O'Leary 1974; Richardson 1975; Stein and Bailey 1973). The fact that married women experience role conflict is well documented in the literature (Cartwright 1978; Hall 1975; Herman and Gyllstrom 1977; Peterson-Hardt and Burlin 1979; Robison 1978; Stake 1979).

In her 1978 study of women physicians, L. Cartwright found that one-half of the sample experienced some strain in integrating professional and home roles, while reporting high career satisfaction. Wives in this sample reduced career involvement in order to reduce stress in relations with husbands. The author cited three factors that account for the stress:

1. Fragmentation: the participation in two areas of life, career and family, that make competing demands on time and energy. In addition to stress, this could also cause overload.
2. Internal conflict: the conflicting expectations that a woman should "act like a woman" and give the needs of her family priority, while at the same time feel the need to "act like a man" and give career goals priority.
3. A nonsupportive environment: this represents the difficulty that women (especially those in male-dominated professions) have in finding support among their peers.

An interesting aspect of this study is the author's suggestion that female physicians are able to tolerate role conflict because of the high levels of gratification they receive from their work. It is of note here that the ability to enact multiple and demanding roles has been found to depend on how greatly the roles are valued (Marks 1977). This would support Richardson's (1981) premise that the degree of role conflict is likely to be influenced by the role context. The implication is that women in less satisfying and less socially valued positions will experience greater difficulty in dealing with multiple roles than those whose work yields greater intrinsic and extrinsic rewards; however, as Richardson (1981) also pointed out, research has shown that high-level occupations tend to demand greater commitment. The demand for greater career involvement that often accompanies the kinds of work from which greater satisfaction can be derived leads to higher levels of strain for some multiple-role negotiators (Pleck 1977).

It appears that whether women are high-achieving professionals or "pink collar" employees for whom work is often just a job (Howe 1977), multiple-role negotiation cannot be accomplished without some degree of role strain. It might be expected that women who are less career involved will be most affected by the time management and role overload aspects of multiple-role negotiation, while women who are in positions demanding greater investment—but also yielding higher satisfaction—will be more affected by the role conflict that results from competing commitment demands of occupation and family.

Of note here is that almost 80 percent of the female work force is employed in nonmanagerial and nonprofessional capacities ("The Superwoman Squeeze" 1980). This would seem to indicate that high levels of stress associated with role overload can be expected among the general population of employed women who are married and/or raising children.

Why are women so underrepresented in the professions and in high-status jobs in business and industry? A study by Peterson-Hardt and Burlin (1979) indicated that the additional responsibilities of familial roles for women influence against high levels of professional involvement.

It is important to realize that while the effects of the women's movement have snowballed during the last decade, adult women in contemporary society grew up with essentially different values from the ones being popularly expressed today. Women who grew up in the post-World War II 1950s, today's 30- to 40-year-olds, were raised during a time when women left the work force to have "2.7 children." These women were lured out of employment by a society that needed jobs for its returning soldiers. The role of homemaker was glorified with renewed fervor.

Certainly, the growing-up experience in the 1950s did not encourage women's involvement in careers outside the home. Women who are products of this experience and who are now involved in careers may have increased difficulty dealing with role conflict, because values internalized in childhood do not support their need to spend time and energy on professions, sometimes at the expense of their families. Working women who are past the age of 40 are likely to have grown up with even more rigid boundaries concerning appropriate female behavior. When these women work, the work is not viewed as a career, but as a supplement to their husbands' income (Bailyn 1970).

Women who grew up with highly valued domestic roles with little attention paid to careers also tend to impede their own career advancement by creating stressful situations caused by conflict (Whitfield 1978). These women attempt to function in their domestic role as fully as they did before they were working (Stake 1979). Stein and Bailey (1973) stated that this is a physically and emotionally exhausting way of living, which does not facilitate career success. It has been shown that some women would rather overload their own role assignments than upset the status quo of division of labor in the home (Berkove 1979).

Dual-Career Couples and Domestic Division of Labor

In his 1979 study of married women returning to school, Berkove found that the wife's increased responsibilities outside the home had little effect on division of tasks within the home. Wives reported increases stress from the increased responsibilities (role overload). Other research confirms that while women are engaging in more outside activities, men have not engaged in a corresponding redistribution of household responsibility (Beckman and Houser 1979; Berger et al. 1977; Berkove 1979; Booth 1979; Richardson 1975; Robison 1978). Pleck (1979) was optimistic that men will gradually become increasingly involved in family roles in response to women's increased participation in the labor force. The reality, however, is different. While men have increased their awareness that they are capable of more expanded family roles, they have continued to avoid taking them on in addition to their already highly valued career role (Moreland and Schwebel 1982).

It can be speculated that wives' overload, coupled with nonsupport from husbands, is a potential source of tension in dual-career marriages. It appears that some women have avoided this possible area of tension and have reduced the negative influences of role conflict on their careers by sacrificing the more traditional feminine role in favor of the career mode.

Limitation of Social Roles

A study of academic and professional employees in a university setting (Herman and Gyllstrom 1977) found that women experienced greater degrees of conflict between work and home maintenance roles than their male colleagues. Apparently, many of these women resolved some of the conflict by remaining single. The study reported twice as many unmarried women in the sample across all job classifications as unmarried men. A study done ten years earlier (Simon, Clark, and Galway 1967) on a sample of doctoral degree holders found that 95 percent of men with doctorates were married, compared with 50 percent of the women.

The implication of both studies is that men can—and do—have both marriage and a career, but that women who place high value on a career may tend to limit their social roles (Mueller and Campbell 1977). The similarity of the studies is worth noting, especially because one was conducted in 1967, before the effects of the women's liberation movement, and the other was conducted in 1977, when the movement was a major social influence.

It has been shown that women experience much higher levels of role strain than men, a fact that can account for men's ability to combine work and family roles. This is largely because the primacy of a man's role as wage earner is socially recognized, while a woman's role as wage earner must coexist with her traditional priority role of wife and mother. There is evidence that the additional responsibility of having children further increases stress and conflict for multiple-role women (Hall 1975; Orden and Bradburn 1969; Robison 1978; Stake 1979).

Balancing Career and Motherhood

As we stated earlier, 43 percent of employed women have children under the age of six. These women are likely to experience higher degrees of role overload than married women without children because child care is added to their household tasks. If these women have internalized guilt feelings over the amount of time they spend away from their children, they will also experience higher degrees of role conflict and associated stress. This guilt is an outgrowth of popular acceptance of the idea in U.S. society that there is such a thing as "the perfect mother" (Wilborn 1976).

There is a widespread belief that the quality of mothering is responsible for every aspect of a child's growth and development. Given this widely accepted premise, it is easy to understand why women who combine careers and motherhood suffer a great deal of stress over whether or not their dual role has adverse effects on their children. In addition, the amount of conflict caused by balancing career and motherhood roles is likely to have considerable influence on birthrate patterns.

Multiple Roles and Fertility

A study conducted by Beckman (1978) showed that professional women were likely to consider that having children interfered with employment. The study supported the concept that high role conflict is associated with lower fertility. Two other studies, one with college seniors (Altman and Grossman 1977) and the other with graduate students (Farley 1970), have implications for future trends in female fertility patterns. In both samples the majority of women expressed the belief that having children would interfere with career achievement.

Also noteworthy are the large numbers of women who have delayed childbearing into their thirties in exchange for career development (U.S., National Center for Health Statistics 1981) but who do plan to have children. A study reported in the New England Journal of Medicine (DeCherney and Berkowitz 1982) clearly established that female fertility greatly decreases in women over 30 years of age. Such medical evidence may influence some women to choose a younger age for childbearing and, consequently, to delay career advancement if they wish to avoid negotiating multiple roles. Or the evidence may force women who clearly choose career as first priority to give up the idea of having a family at some future time.

We have seen that social changes during the last 20 years have created new options for women; they also have created new issues. One major change is that many women have given up the notion that their life cycle must center around the family life cycle. For many women, the traditional role of wife/homemaker/mother has been expanded to include a career outside the home. The increased responsibilities resulting from the expanded role have caused conflict and overload. The expanded role has affected relationships between women and men and has influenced women's childbearing patterns. There is some evidence that the roles of wife/mother and worker are—or are perceived to be—at odds with each other, and that an investment in one results in a concomitant reduction of success or perceived reduction of success in the other.

Problems of conflict, overload, coping, and time management reflect one side of the effects of women's expanded roles. The beneficial aspects of women's expanded roles are felt by women, men, and society. In order to achieve a more balanced view of the issues women face in multiple-role negotiation, the positive aspects of expanded roles must be explored.

WOMEN'S SELF-ESTEEM AND MENTAL HEALTH

Although research has indicated that many women experience conflict about the dual role of wife/career women and that this conflict can reduce career commitment and achievement, women working outside the home report high levels of happiness and self-esteem (Hall and Gordon 1973; Heckman, Bryson, and Bryson 1977; Hiller and Philliber 1978; Robison 1978). It can be speculated that satisfaction would be even higher if role conflict and overload could be reduced.

Research has shown that women's traditional, narrowly defined roles have caused higher levels of frustration and dissatisfaction for them (Gove and Tudor 1972). This has contributed to greater degrees of mental illness among women than men (Chesler 1972). Less-restricted women's roles and more opportunities for internal and external rewards could reduce this phenomenon (Robison 1978) if improved methods of coping with role strain are developed.

MARITAL SATISFACTION

As we have noted previously, role overload and unequal distribution of domestic tasks within a marriage have the potential to negatively affect the marital relationship. On the other hand, research has indicated that a woman's freedom to choose among alternative life-styles is an important predictor of marital happiness (Order and Bradburn 1969).

Higher levels of marital satisfaction are perceived by husbands of working wives. Separate studies by Booth (1979) and Robison (1978) found that husbands of employed women are happier and under less stress than husbands of housewives. This is due in part to decreased financial pressure and the husband's perception that his wife is happier because she is working (Heckman, Bryson, and Bryson 1977). It has also been found that even when a wife's occupational achievement is higher than her husband's, the husband's marital satisfaction is not reduced (Richardson 1979).

EFFECTS ON CHILDREN

Despite the fact that multiple-role women suffer conflict about dividing their child-care responsibilities with career activities, two authors have indicated that a mother's employment outside the home does not have adverse effects on children (Etaugh 1980; Hoffman 1979). As a matter of fact, Hoffman stated that women's involvement in careers outside the home will have long-range positive effects on their children. She contends that multiple-role models are better than one and that children with mothers who work are likely to grow up to be more independent and better able to cope with the multiple roles that society will inevitably expect from them. Because the research findings of the effects of maternal employment on children are inconclusive (Smith 1981), it might be well for working mothers to accept Hoffman's optimistic opinion in order to better cope with some aspects of role conflict.

SOCIAL BENEFITS OF WOMEN'S EXPANDED ROLES

Women's career participation brings a wealth of new talent and abilities to the labor force. In addition, the expansion of women's roles into the work world should gradually free men to invest some of their energies in the family system (Pleck 1979). This liberation of both men and women to develop multiple dimensions of themselves should have widespread positive effects on society as a whole.

The positive aspects of women's multiple roles are great, and they can be further enhanced by reduction of the conflict and stress that hamper negotiation of these roles. Social change is necessary to provide a more supportive atmosphere for women to expand their roles beyond the narrow confines of wife/mother, so that they can more freely participate in activities outside the home.

REFERENCES

Altman, S. I., and F. K. Grossman. 1977. "Women's Career Plans and Maternal Employment." Psychology of Women Quarterly 1(4): 365–77.

Bailyn, L. 1970. "Career and Family Orientations of Husbands and Wives in Relation to Marital Happiness." Human Relations 23(2): 97–114.

Beckman, L. J. 1978. "The Relative Rewards and Costs of Parenthood and Employment for Employed Women." Psychology of Women Quarterly 2(3): 215–33.

Beckman, L. J., and B. B. Houser. 1979. "The More You Have the More You Do: The Relationship between Wife's Employment, Sex-Role, Attitudes, and Household Behavior." Psychology of Women Quarterly 4(2): 160–74.

Berger, M., B. S. Wallston, M. Foster, and L. Wright. 1977. "You and Me against the World: Dual Career Couples and Joint Job Seeking." Journal of Research and Development in Education 10: 30–37.

Berkove, G. F. 1979. "Perceptions of Husband Support by Returning Women Students." Family Coordinator 28: 451-57.

Booth, A. 1979. "Does Wives' Employment Cause Stress for Husbands?" Family Coordinator 28: 445-49.

Cartwright, L. K. 1978. "Career Satisfaction and Role Harmony in
a Sample of Young Women Physicians." Journal of Vocational
Behavior 12: 184-96.

Chesler, P. 1972. Women and Madness. New York: Doubleday.

DeCherney, A. H., and G. S. Berkowitz. 1982. "Female Fecundity
and Age." New England Journal of Medicine 306(7): 424-26.

Etaugh, C. 1980. "Effects of Non-maternal Care on Children: Research Evidence and Popular Views." American Psychologist
35: 309-19.

Farley, J. 1970. "Graduate Women: Career Aspirations and Desired Family Size." American Psychologist 25: 1099-1100.

Fitzgerald, L. F., and J. O. Crites. 1980. "Toward a Career
Psychology of Women: What Do We Need to Know?" Journal of
Counseling Psychology 27: 44-62.

Goode, W. J. 1960. "A Theory of Role Strain." American Sociological Review 25: 483-96.

Gove, W. R., and J. F. Tudor. 1973. "Adult Sex Roles and Mental
Illness." American Journal of Sociology 78(4): 813-35.

Hall, D. T. 1975. "Pressures from Work, Self, and Home in the
Life Stages of Married Women." Journal of Vocational Behavior
6: 121-32.

Hall, D. T., and F. E. Gordon. 1973. "Career Choices of Married
Women: Effects on Conflict, Role Behavior and Satisfaction."
Journal of Applied Psychology 58(1): 42-48.

Harmon, L. W. 1970. "Anatomy of Career Commitment in Women."
Journal of Counseling Psychology 17: 77-80.

Heckman, N. A., R. Bryson, and J. B. Bryson. 1977. "Problems
of Professional Couples: A Content Analysis." Journal of Marriage and the Family 39: 323-30.

Herman, J. B., and K. K. Gyllstrom. 1977. "Working Men and Women: Inter- and Intra-role Conflict." Psychology of Women Quarterly 1(4): 319-33.

Hiller, D. A., and W. W. Philliber. 1978. "The Derivation of Status Benefits from Occupational Attainments of Working Wives." Journal of Marriage and the Family 40: 63-68.

Hoffman, L. W. 1979. "Changes in Family Roles, Socialization and Sex Differences." American Psychologist 32: 644-57.

Hooper, J. O. 1979. "My Wife, the Student." Family Coordinator 28: 459-64.

Howe, L. 1977. Pink Collar Workers. New York: G. P. Putnam's Sons.

Marks, S. R. 1977. "Multiple Roles and Role Strain: Some Notes on Human Energy, Time and Commitment." American Sociological Review 42: 921-36.

Moreland, J., and A. I. Schwebel. 1982. "A Gender Role Transcendent Perspective on Fathering." Counseling Psychologist 9(4): 45-53.

Mueller, C. W., and B. G. Campbell. 1977. "Female Occupational Achievement and Marital Status: A Research Note." Journal of Marriage and the Family 39: 587-93.

O'Leary, V. E. 1974. "Some Attitudinal Barriers to Occupational Aspirations in Women." Psychological Bulletin 81(11): 809-26.

O'Neil, J. M. 1981. "Male Sex-Role Conflicts, Sexism and Masculinity: Psychological Implications for Men, Women and the Counseling Psychologist." Counseling Psychologist 9(2): 61-81.

Orden, R. R., and N. M. Bradburn. 1969. "Working Wives and Marriage Happiness." American Journal of Sociology 74: 392-407.

Peterson-Hardt, S., and F. D. Burlin. 1979. "Sex Differences in Perceptions of Familial and Occupational Roles." Journal of Vocational Behavior 14: 316-16.

Pleck, J. H. 1979. "Men's Family Work: Three Perspectives and Some New Data." Family Coordinator 28(4): 481-95.

_____. 1977. "The Work Family Role System." Social Problems 24: 417-27.

Richardson, J. G. 1979. "Wife Occupational Superiority and Marital Troubles: An Examination of the Hypothesis." Journal of Marriage and the Family 41: 63-71.

Richardson, M. S. 1981. "Occupational and Family Roles: A Neglected Intersection." Counseling Psychologist 9(4): 13-23.

_____. 1975. "Self-Concepts and Role Concepts in the Career Orientation of College Women." Journal of Counseling Psychology 22(2): 122-26.

Robison, E. 1978. "Strain and Dual Role Occupation among Women." Ph.D. dissertation, City University of New York. Dissertation Abstracts International 38A.

Scarato, A. M., and B. A. Sigall. 1979. "Multiple Role Women." Counseling Psychologist 8(1): 26-27.

Simon, R. J., S. M. Clark, and K. Galway. 1967. "The Woman Ph.D.: A Recent Profile." Social Problems 15(2): 221-36.

Smith, E. J. 1981. "The Working Mother: A Critique of the Research." Journal of Vocational Behavior 19: 191-211.

Stake, J. E. 1979. "Women's Self Estimates of Competence and the Resolution of the Career/Home Conflict." Journal of Vocational Behavior 14: 33-42.

Stein, A. H., and M. M. Bailey. 1973. "The Socialization of Achievement Orientation in Females." Psychological Bulletin 80(5): 345-65.

"The Superwoman Squeeze." 1980. Newsweek, May 19, pp. 72-79.

U.S., Department of Commerce, Bureau of the Census. 1979. Population Profile of the United States: 1978, Population Characteristics (Current Population Reports, Series P-20, no. 336). Washington, D.C.: Government Printing Office.

U.S., National Center for Health Statistics. 1981. Advance Report of the Natality Statistics, 1979 (Monthly Viral Statistics Report 30[6], Supplement). Washington, D.C.: Government Printing Office.

Van Dusen, R. A., and E. B. Sheldon. 1976. "The Changing Status of American Women: A Life Cycle Perspective." American Psychologist 31: 106-15.

Whitfield, M. D. 1978. "Stresses Associated with Career Success for Women." Canadian Psychiatric Association Journal 23: 9-14.

Wilborn, B. L. 1976. "The Myth of the Perfect Mother." Counseling Psychologist 6(2): 42-45.

Wolfson, K. P. 1976. "Career Development Patterns of College Women." Journal of Counseling Psychology 23: 119-25.

3

The Mid-life
Crisis in Women

Margot Tallmer

The term <u>mid-life crisis</u> has assumed a certain psychological cachet. Gould (1980) suggested that the pervasive popularization of the phenomenon may actually reflect a need on the part of writers and analysts to explain their own age-related intrapsychic difficulties within the framework of an acceptable, nonthreatening label. The crisis is popularly thought of as a period for appraising one's life situation, assessing both past losses and potential roots for dealing with the remainder of life—a life now seen as more than half over. It has been suggested that we define <u>mid-life</u> as age 35, in order to separate mid-life from menopause. One-half of a woman's life-span would actually be closer to age 38 or 39, nearly ten years before menopause.

To comprehend any individual's mid-life crisis and the effects of age-related losses, one must know if the person being considered is male or female. In this chapter, general role differences between the sexes are considered and specific female changes are examined, that is, the ending of the menstrual cycle (a biological event) and the departure of the children from the home (an occurrence causing psychological shifts). These two major changes are designated as integral in theoretical writings and as the factors seen to cause female psychic distress. Symptoms used as evidence of their negative potential include depression, frequent use of medication, and high frequency of visits to doctors and psychologists. Both major changes are integral parts of the female mid-life crisis; both generally take place at about the same time. The two phenomena also interact.

As late as 1963, when Cumming and Henry were developing disengagement theory (a theory supposedly explaining the withdrawal of the elderly from society), they assumed that women's passage through the life cycle was a smoother route than the one traversed by men. Their explanation? Pivotal roles of homemakers and nurturers continued throughout the female life, while aging male counterparts were obliged to confront critical life alterations, such as retirement. The work role is seen as central to the lives of men, occupying the most role space and offering the greatest social as well as monetary rewards. The female labor role is less consistently and clearly defined.

More sophisticated research has suggested that, contrariwise, role discontinuity is a major characteristic and a central adaptation of a woman's life. Role shifts and vocational changes, mandated by interruptions for childbearing, husband's career, and consequent geographical shifts, and the caring for elderly parents all demand a large amount of flexibility. (Actually, this flexibility is of great service in successful aging.) Further evidence of role changes for women is the fact that the spouse role disappears far more often in the case of women than men; in 70 percent of widowhood states, the survivor is a woman. Thus, women can adjust better because they have been obliged to do so often, and a lifetime of contradictory roles and conflicting demands becomes a positive experience. Mulvey (1963) confirmed that high satisfaction for women obtains from reentry into a previously abandoned career decision or a career that had been temporarily put aside, plus volunteer activities, or a lifetime split between working and homemaking. The least happy woman had adhered to one job, either homemaking or outside work. Perhaps mere change qua change is satisfying and growth producing, or it may be argued that the mastery of new skills and adaptations required of women yields satisfaction. Questions easily surface: Were the changes voluntary? Did the women see the alterations as helpful to their husbands or to their families or to themselves? Do women hold back on total commitment, knowing that changes are likely? Permanence is less often a characteristic of a woman's life.

According to Kutner's theory of the social nature of aging (1961), we are obliged throughout life to adjust to novel situations, to establish new plateaus, and to realign our goals, defenses, and strategies. Women should excel at this because they have performed the tasks so frequently. It should be noted that the changes we are considering here are not truly voluntary; the menopause is time-specified, biologically dictated, and the empty nest syndrome is fairly well determined by external forces. It is also relevant to stress that the phrase "loss of role" is an unfair designation, for women do continue in roles as homemakers, mothers, and daughters, with each role modified, perceived differently, and component parts shifted. What is really being discussed are role changes as well as role losses.

Demographic changes have also illuminated the complex life patterns of women: namely, the diminution of time typically spent in child rearing and the consequent extended period without children in

the home; more free time because of labor-saving devices; a length-
ened period alone as a widow; the high rise in divorce rates; a growth
in single-by-choice statistics; increasing educational levels that post-
pone marriage; voluntary childlessness; and the high inflation rate
that sends many women out to work.

Deutsch (1944-45) saw termination of the menses as the most
trying time in the life of a woman, and many others have agreed that
it is an important rite de passage that ushers in a host of physical
symptoms for most women. Symptoms range from minor ones (hot
flashes) to acutely serious ones (depression is the most serious and
frequent). Although many stress the potential for sublimation in a
wide variety of previously restricted activities during this period,
there persist strongly held, widespread negative conceptions about
menopause. For example, in the library the word is indexed under
"female diseases." The stereotype is of a difficult period, both biologically and psychologically. Thus, it may come as a jolt to many
that menopausal women regard themselves far more favorably than
do others; that is, they recognize the possibility of difficulties but
themselves experience a persistent and sustained feeling of well-being
(Neugarten 1970). Menopause appears to be less of a topic for personal discussion than other female biological events such as the onset
of menstruation. There is no particular commercial or media ex-
ploitation of menopause. The phenomenon itself is not an observable
one like pregnancy. Perhaps it is a task of female psychoanalysts or
psychologists to attempt an understanding, as they themselves must
be affected in some ways by their mothers' waning fertility at the time
of their own greatest reproductive potential. For many analysts,
menopause and its putative difficulties reflect a continued lack of
oedipal resolution. Certainly, the now infertile menopausal female
may be perceived as sexually less threatening, older, and less eroti-
cally attractive. Incidentally, women are perceived as being old at
younger ages throughout life than are men, and they are thus endowed
with negative characteristics of old age at an earlier time in the life
cycle. With consideration given to the extra years of their life-span,
they are "aged" for a disproportionate length of time. Women are
old much longer than men are old.

In a further refinement of Freudian notions of the oedipal conflict, Lebe (1982) suggested that its resolution must include the separation from the early mother object, an object perceived as omnipotent and threatening as well as life-sustaining. Female adult achievement in varied areas, such as school, marriage, and volunteer work,
enhances self-esteem and helps to overcome feelings of inadequacy
engendered by the absence of a penis. By adulthood, then, the woman
is more capable of a realistic perception of men, a perception that
recognizes male requisites for affirmation, achievement, power, and

protection. These drives in men have often forced a repression of af-
fectional relational needs and emotional responsivity. In an important
way, because a female's feared ability to castrate men has not been
confirmed, she can then permit herself vaginal possession of the
phallus without guilt or fear of punishment. She is thus free to channel energy to outside achievement at a time of high biological strength.
When no longer worrying about conception, she can experience sex
for its mutual pleasure rather than as a procreative act. Nurturing
needs will be partially met by grandparenting, a less strenuous, more
voluntary, and more time-limited relationship than mothering. If
this nurturing need is endowed with high superego value for women,
it may contribute to difficulty in the work arena, where competition
and nonnurturing activities are important. In fact, work activities
themselves may be seen as conflicting with the nurturing role.

Both menopause and the empty nest have served as facile explanations for female psychiatric disturbances despite the empirical
evidence to the contrary (Campbell, Converse, and Rodgers 1976;
Lowenthal 1975; Maas and Kuypers 1974; McKinley and Jeffries 1974;
Neugarten 1968). Thinking seems to follow a particular pattern:
women's centrality is her biological potential. It follows naturally
that the aborting of such an important capability—that is, the ability
to procreate—inevitably leads to distress. Work or voluntary activities can be only restitutive. Motherhood is publicly heralded, in
sharp contrast to menopause, and is regarded as a major positive
psychological and biological milestone, invested with many intrapsychic meanings. The more obvious meanings include the culmination
of a sexual act, the opportunity for vicarious rebirth and a second
chance at one's own life, the reversal of roles experienced with one's
own parents, the extraordinarily intimate relationship with another
human being who is at first helpless but who represents at the same
time one's own helplessness, one's own mortality, and even one's
potential immortality. Analytic formations include the familiar
Freudian equation of penis equals child, that is, women compensate
for their phallic minuses by birthing. However, motherhood is not a
unitary phenomenon nor does it retain the same significance for the
person throughout her life. In mid-life, children generally leave
home.

The empty nest syndrome has been described as "a mother's
depressive reaction to the loss of children. . . . A connection between her identity as a mother and her ego-ideal is disrupted; the
self-esteem is damaged, and the ensuing anger and her strenuous
defensive reaction against this rage temporarily paralyze efforts to
shift to other facets of her valued identity" (Avery 1981).

The loss of being a full-time mother is seen as serious, but
other developmental events and variables affect that loss or even pre-

vent negative effects from appearing at all. After the departure of
the children, we empirically witness that daily life becomes much
less complicated. Even a home where the family is gone all day has
been charged through the years with the presence of others. Those
others, adolescent children, have often activated a good deal of family
tension as they struggled loudly and unpredictably toward autonomy.
Their leave-taking can be of enormous relief to many women, particularly if these offspring function well, causing positive appraisals to
accrue to the parents. If they do not fare well, there is still the
daily comfort of no longer being totally responsible for their activities
and actions. Out of sight, somewhat out of mind and worry. Many
teenagers are also sources of competitive envy, blessed as they are
by seemingly infinite vigor, attractiveness, and youth. To the extent
the parents feel inadequate or insufficient themselves, the evoked
potential for envy rises proportionately, negatively impacting upon
family relationships.

A rather current addition to the customary intergenerational
strain is the pronounced deemphasis on the home arena, with a
woman continuing to identify with her spouse and depending upon him
to control her destructive urges. Should no channel for aggressive
impulses be available (the husband may die or shun the burden of home),
some women may experience depression (Gutmann 1980). For other
women, a time for self-examination and development has arrived, reinforced by the heightened awareness of mortality. Women may be
particularly alert to death concerns, having had the constant responsibility for young children and, often, the caretaking of older parents.
Being alone is restorative, the famous "room of one's own," and it
permits self-exploration. The burdens of being central to a family's
interaction—experiencing herself as (1) ever open to interruptions by
others who require responsiveness and constant emotional sensitivity
and (2) responsible for the inexorable daily tasks need to mechanically
maintain family life—are diminished, and the diminution may be a welcome one. Although mothering continues, it does so on a less intense
basis. While this must connote a certain loss of power, since a mother
plays such an important role in the child's early life, the gain resides
in the knowledge that all of one's actions are not so fraught with consequences. Women who thought of no other life plan than motherhood
and being a wife are now free to consider other alternatives. If a
variety of roles become possible and a societal imprimatur is con-
ferred upon them, middle-aged women may select from manifold options and substitute one commitment for another. This change comes
at a time that is much earlier than a man's retirement at age 65. In
passing, it should be noted that the current group of mid-life females
may have to face the greatest difficulties as they try to navigate between the liberating pronouncements of the women's movement and
the traditional matriarchal role.

A final question: What if there is no empty nest syndrome because there was no nest? Gutmann's intriguing finding of female patients suffering for the first time from depression or transient psychoses sheds another dimension on motherhood (1980). This sample had a disproportionate share of childless women—childless for varying psychological and biological reasons. Following the death of their own aged mothers or subsequent to a serious illness, they became unusually vulnerable to late-life depression and transient psychosis, phenomena that occur often after the death of a mother or the diagnosis of a potentially fatal disease in themselves. Having a child evidently permits a maturation that includes a final separation from the maternal object and the acceptance of the finite life cycle. Childless women have never experienced the great transformation of narcissism that renders the child's life more precious than their own. Accordingly, they remain disastrously vulnerable to the late-life intimations of mortality. It is better to have loved and lost. Thus, Gutmann felt that motherhood obliges one to confront her mortality and to decisively separate from the maternal object.

Empirically, one can witness Gutmann's belief that mothers fear greatly that they will predecease their children. Folklore states that one can never get over the death of a child. It is the quintessential horror. Such a shift in one's narcissism to the child leads to a yielding of one's centrality, one's omnipotence. But having a child does not seem to force necessarily the severing of early ties to the maternal object. Clinical settings handle many cases of women who are still unable to separate from the mother despite having children of their own. Perhaps the woman is less open to depressed psychological functioning after motherhood because she feels she has satisfied society's traditional goals, is supported by her offspring, has matured through having children, or has derived from them great satisfaction and high self-esteem that continues to accrue to her as they prosper. Having children, once considered woman's occupation, must be studied within the historical context.

In summary, I have suggested that pathological mourning prompted by menopause and the children's leaving home has distorted the public perception of these happenings and has focused and limited attention to the deviant as rationalization for ageist and sexist thinking. As with any other psychic event, these two phenomena must be defined and interpreted differently for each individual. The majority of women apparently traverse this period of life in terms of crisis theory. The resolution of any crisis can enhance life satisfaction with opportunities for growth and expansion. The prism of stereotyped thinking about the female life cycle distorts our perceptions and precludes examination of the more authentic causes of depression and dissatisfaction in late-life women.

REFERENCES

Avery, N. 1981. "Phallic Narcissistic Vulnerability and the Empty Nest." Journal of American Academy of Psychoanalysis 9(4): 525-37.

Campbell, A., P. E. Converse, and W. L. Rodgers. 1976. The Quality of American Life. New York: Russell Sage Foundation.

Cumming, E., and W. E. Henry. 1963. Growing Old. New York: Basic Books.

Deutsch, H. 1944-45. The Psychology of Women. New York: Grune & Stratton.

Gould, R. L. 1980. "Transformational Tasks in Adulthood." In Adulthood and the Aging Process, edited by S. L. Greenspan and G. H. Pollock, pp. 55-89. Bethesda, Md.: National Institute of Mental Health.

Gutmann, D. 1980. "Psychoanalysis and Aging: A Developmental View. The Course of Life: Psychoanalytic Contributions toward Understanding Personality Development." In Adulthood and the Aging Process, edited by S. L. Greenspan and G. H. Pollock, pp. 489-517. Bethesda, Md.: National Institute of Mental Health.

Kutner, B. 1961. "The Social Nature of Aging." Paper presented at the meeting of the American Psychological Association, New York.

Lebe, D. 1982. "Individuation of Women." Psychoanalytic Review 69(1): 63-74.

Lowenthal, M. 1975. "Psychosocial Variations across the Adult Life Course: Frontiers for Research and Policy." Gerontologist 15: 6-12.

Maas, H., and J. Kuypers. 1974. From Thirty to Seventy: A Forty-Year Longitudinal Study of Adult Life Styles and Personality. San Francisco: Jossey-Bass.

McKinley, S., and M. Jeffries. 1974. "The Menopausal Syndrome." Journal of Preventive Social Medicine 28(2): 108-15.

Mulvey, M. C. 1963. "Psychological and Sociological Factors in Prediction of Career Patterns of Women." Genetic Psychological Monographs, no. 68.

Neugarten, B. L. 1970. "Dynamics of Transition of Middle Age to Old Age: Adaptation and the Life Cycle." Psychiatry 4: 71.

_____. 1968. Middle Age and Aging. Chicago: University of Chicago Press.

4

Women, Aging, and Loss: The Gain Factor

Marcella Bakur Weiner
and
Marion Adler

Women have been indoctrinated with a minus theory of development. As with all indoctrination, concepts are internalized and then
become part of the stored material used in self-fulfillment or nonful-
fillment. Women are tied to their destiny of loss—ending in death,
the final loss or surrender of self. When it is related to positive or
life-enhancing concepts, female sexuality, with its inherent life-force
properties, becomes tied to "issues" (a theoretical abstraction), not
to "woman" (a feeling, living, human being). Although it is not inten-
tional, we nonetheless perpetuate the myth of woman as facing and
succumbing to the inevitable losses thrust upon her from early years
on.

This belief has a long and prestigious history. Based upon one
of Freud's central postulates, it states that the resolution of the oedipal or the "positive oedipal" in females can only develop as a consequence of the castration complex (Fliegel 1982). Implicit in this
theory is that the little girl really begins as a little boy, desiring a
penis in order to be able to have coitus with the mother. Granted his
profound contributions and influence, Freud was not the only one to
see woman as negative in nature. Deutsch, in speaking of narcissism,
passivity, and masochism as being essential to woman's nature, saw
the former as a pathological overemphasis on physical beauty and as
compensatory for the self-esteem that lack of a penis assigns her to
(Lachman 1982). Perhaps there is still a pervasive belief, masked
in rhetoric and seemingly liberated slogans, that female anatomy is
the major barrier to culturally valued achievements.

Despite the ingrained images of woman as less than man, the
literature and empirical observation point to the fact that woman is
at least an equal partner. For example, Freud's theory of oedipal
resolution in the female is unsupported by clinical data from child

analyses; that is, it is suggested that the early phallic phase is not negative oedipal for the girl and positive oedipal for the boy, but that this stage is merely narcissistic for both sexes. It is further pointed out that girl/boy identity emerges in the symbiotic phase. For the girl this necessary identity (or ability to attach oneself to another) continues, so that later her task appears to be the ability to establish her separateness. In contrast, the boy, attempting to establish gender identity, is seen as more vulnerable and "laden with conflict" (Fliegel 1982). Symbiosis is seen to be easier for the infant girl, in that the larger size of the male child and his tendency toward more movement may make him more difficult to soothe and may shorten a needed symbiosis with the parenting figure. This ability for early attachment, sustained over a period of time as intrinsic to a developmental stage, is noted as essential for later development. Heinz Kohut (1977) emphasized that the child retains the mother as a self-object, gradually to be internalized and fixed as a psychic structure. This psychic structure, according to Kohut, is the very foundation of the "self," a blending of self-object relationships, which gives the person the sense of self-cohesion and self-esteem so essential to successful living. Most important, it is this self, now a hypothesized structure, that is the major resource to be used many years later when, as adults, we deal with the losses implicit in life's experiences and our own aging. For even where loss of a loved person takes place—an unavoidable occurrence that no one escapes—and depression or mourning follows, it is suggested that it is not the actual missing person who is mourned but, rather, "the missing segments of the psychic structure": a part of that self developed as a consequence of early attachment to a loving figure, which is now a valued image within oneself. This self is truly mourned (Weiner and White 1983). This self, developed over time, also contains the roots of our core identity, which, despite the continuous changes in our life, allows for sameness. This self-continuity is the repository for all early ideas, thoughts, feelings, and memories, stored for later exploration in life's quieter times—or as aging becomes more visible and predominant.

The early and extended symbiosis may be critical to the aging woman. Society has long dichotomized male/female roles; sociological theory spoke of the male's role being highly instrumental, the woman's more affective or expressive. "She," it has been said, "feels," while he is busy "doing." Man was concerned with achieving, having power, and becoming an autonomous human being. Woman was the nurturer. Valued and devalued, woman was valued as a caretaker, helpmate, weaver of and active participant in caring relationships; she was devalued as being too dependent. Tied to others in an overlong symbiosis, she is said to never fully achieve separateness, her own personal autonomy at best a shadowy substance. Her giving, conceded to be life-sustaining, is nonetheless seen as weakness rather than strength (Gilligan 1982). Yet, contradictions abound. Women are survivors in terms of longevity, and the more dominant the woman (possibly the more assertive and with a strong sense of self), the more successfully does she age (Neugarten 1968). Considered intuitive, she instinctively reaches out, valuing intimacy, relationships, and caring; men, it is said, have to learn them.

This natural committing of oneself to another may be a link to survivorship in women, for it is they who have that confidante or intimate-other deemed essential to later life. The male, depending only upon one female for his intimacy needs, may appear bereft of a network when she dies and, as has been noted, may die soon afterward (Botwinick 1979). Conversely, perhaps women's sense of self, which is woven out of the fiber of early, continuous attachment to the mothering person, persists, as does her ability to maintain affiliations. Disruptions or losses of others may then be perceived as losses of parts of the self.

This may appear in other disruptions of life such as marital divorce or separation. Where this does occur in later life, women report more agitation than men, despite the fact that men experience a lower sense of overall well-being (Chiriboga 1982). It is interesting that despite this greater emotional upheaval, the older woman, upon actual divorce or separation, shows an improvement in health status. It is possible that despite chaos arising out of the shifting of parts of the psychic structure called the self, compensatory mechanisms of a substantial nature take over and predominate. This phenomenon may also reflect the closure needed by many women to end what had been perceived to be a poor marriage. This sense of closure, or completeness of a stage, may be the primary soother of experienced hurts and disappointments.

Loneliness, too, may be the consequence of perceived losses. A recent Danish study showed that the feeling of loneliness increased from 12 percent at 62 years of age to 23 percent at 72 years of age (Berg et al. 1981). However, a national Swedish study showed that 20 percent of people between the ages of 60 and 65 felt lonely, while the proportion rose to above 40 percent for those aged 80 and older. Again related to the feeling of loneliness were states of widow/widowerhood and lack of contact with others, in particular children and old friends. The perception of loneliness was more common among women, despite the seeming contradiction that whereas widowerhood narrowed the circle of friends for men, it did not for widows. Noted, too, was that loneliness in both sexes related to neuroticism as defined by the Minnesota Multiphasic Personality Inventory neuroticism scale and symptom checklists. However, it is also possible that measured neuroticism may be a consequence of loneliness, not a cause of it.

While networks appear to be the key for successful aging, recent emphasis has been placed on the quality, not the quantity, of relationships. Thus, although childless widows were more lonely and dissatisfied with their lives and had lower overall well-being than widows with grown children, these differences were minimal compared with the impact of social interaction on general well-being.

Along with the emphasis on relationships with others is a newer focus on a relationship with the self. One author states: "I know of no formal research which conveys the experience of widows actively engaged in interaction with the self as a distinct being." The writer then goes on to state that aging widows in her sample who have been able to meet socioemotional needs by relating to themselves, while not typical, "intrigue and inspire" others with their style of coping. These widows "make themselves the objects of their compassion, nurturance and care." The inference is that the woman who relies upon and turns to her own self in need truly believes she is her own best friend. The quality of this relationship in the later years is one of discovery or, more accurately, rediscovery—the getting to know "someone" better, the sharing in a self-to-self way of the most intimate thoughts and feelings, and most urgently, the finding of a responsive reactor. The author notes that from her observations these widowed women are not full of pathology but, rather, are "alive with energy, able to learn from new experience, and to respond to others. Their self-esteem is high and their joy in living is evident" (Barrett 1981).

Perhaps this relates to the reactivation in later years of self-object images formed from early life on and again brought into play when an emptiness, translated into an actual loss, occurs. At that point in time, it may be that memory traces and pictures within ourselves are brought to the fore to fill the gap created by the loss and to offer newer satisfactions and some joy in living, despite the intensity of the attachment and, therefore, of the loss. Again, as with much of life, it may not be the quantity of early self-object relationships that is most relevant but, rather, the quality, for whatever is stored and reactivated must have profound meaning for the person. Extending the concept of quality past self-self relationships to relationships with others, it is now understood that quality relationships are most often found in the family, despite the myth that Americans are a noncaring people (Weiner, Teresi, and Streich 1983). Daughters, in particular, appear to have a firmer commitment to aging parents than sons, as measured by frequency of contact and performed tasks. Again, it may be the girl's early training in affiliation that persists into the later years, so that when she is in the middle years, she is placed and places herself in a caring relationship with aging parents. Although the female takes on the responsibility for care of aging parents with some reciprocity of tasks and emotional bonds (as more recent research seems to indicate), the older woman caring for her ailing spouse is likely to be twice as much depressed as her counterpart not in this position.* Yet the aging woman persists in her role as caretaker, beginning in the middle years with care of parents and continuing with care of a spouse. Although possibly burdened in both situations, she carries on—and survives.

That the woman more than adequately copes with stress and loss is also demonstrated by newer evidence, which states that it is not the so-called empty nest syndrome that demoralizes women but, rather, the full nest. This newer awareness of the emergence of and pleasure in the reliance upon the self comes as a welcome surprise. For, as has been noted in this chapter, the focus has been on the woman's attachment to others and her overdependence. Only now is it understood that passive dependency in women is not a mature adult state but a partially resolved individuation from the mother, later transferred onto men (Lebe 1982). Yet, if the woman uses her self as a major resource through the natural pulls and pushes of life, the strengths must be there from early years on. Perhaps for her, self-reliance—or more descriptively, self-joy—had always been there, but these self-related qualities were discouraged and rendered invisible.

Self-joy and feats of coping are evident in recent research on sexuality in the later years. In a new study of 800 older people living in the community, women stated that sex lives for them in the later years were the best. The typical older female (average age 70) who did not have a male sex partner suggested well-functioning alternatives such as sublimation, masturbation, sharing of the male, and lesbianism. In responding to the question of why older people do not have sex as often as they would like, both men and women stated, "No partner" (Starr and Weiner 1982). The woman's potential and actual loss of a male partner in the later years is dealt with by suggestions that show the ability to overcome this type of loss. Again the reliance is on either finding satisfaction through others or through masturbation, a turning toward the self for self-pleasure.

In conclusion, if we had to predict what the aging woman would look like in the future, what could we say? Whereas women in the past have had to rely much upon their own personal powers of attractiveness and home-care abilities to attain a sense of achievement, this is no longer true. Women's occupational prestige, recognition,

---

*Personal communication of Barry Gurland's research as related by Jeanne Teresi, Faculty, Geriatrics and Gerontology, Columbia University, New York.

and value for a specific job performance are becoming more of a reality each day. This suggests that women will be less economically dependent in older age because, in retirement, they will have access to monetary benefits not linked to a spouse's pension plans or social security benefits. (Demographic forecasts assume a continuance of the sex differentials in life expectancy, at least into the near future [Abu-Laban 1982].) Should that spouse die, they would not lose dramatically. Furthermore, since a majority of older women may still spend their later years in an unmarried state, the type of preparatory experience engaged in by younger women today may do much to help. When today's younger women are thrust into their own aging, they will more likely have had these kinds of experiences, which would include transitory living/loving relationships, living outside of a traditional marriage, divorce, and more sexual partners than their predecessors. All this experience of coping with beginnings and endings of relationships, with relationships both exploratory and more lasting in nature, may be the ground upon which a more cohesive self and better self-self relationships develop. As one perhaps relies less upon the expectations for self-fulfillment by the other, one can turn more to the expectations and satisfaction of these promises by one's self. Joy can then be found in one's own interior, and the aging woman, trained and performing well her role as giver to others, can finally relax into and experience the pleasure of giving—to her self.

REFERENCES

Abu-Laban, S. M. 1982. "Women and Aging: A Futurist Perspective." Psychology of Women Quarterly 69(1): 63–74.

Barrett, C. J. 1981. "Intimacy in Widowhood." Psychology of Women Quarterly 5(3): 473–85.

Berg, S., et al. 1981. "Loneliness in the Swedish Aged." Journal of Gerontology 36(3): 342–49.

Botwinick, J. 1979. Aging and Behavior. New York: Springer.

Chiriboga, D. A. 1982. "Adaptation to Marital Separation in Later and Earlier Life." Journal of Gerontology 37(1): 109–14.

Fliegel, Z. 1982. "Half a Century Later: Current Status of Freud's Controversial Views on Women." Psychoanalytic Review 69(1): 7–28.

Gilligan, C. 1982. "Why Should a Woman Be More Like a Man?" Psychology Today, June, pp. 68-77.

Kohut, H. 1977. The Restoration of the Self. New York: International Universities Press.

Lachman, F. 1982. "Narcissism and Female Gender Identity: A Reformulation." Psychoanalytic Review 69(1): 43-62.

Lebe, D. 1982. "Individuation of Women." Psychoanalytic Review 69(1): 63-74.

Neugarten, B. 1972. Middle Age and Aging. Chicago: University of Chicago Press.

Starr, B., and M. B. Weiner. 1982. The Starr-Weiner Report on Sex and Sexuality in the Mature Years. New York: McGraw-Hill.

Weiner, M. B., and M. B. White. 1983. "Depression as the Search for the Lost Self." Psychotherapy: Theory, Research, and Practice 19(4): 491-99.

Weiner, M. B., J. Teresi, and C. Streich. 1983. Old People Are a Burden but Not My Parents. New York: Spectrum/Trade.

5

Dynamic Considerations in the Treatment of Grief in the Young Widow and Her Children

Diane Eaton

Catastrophic illness and death of a spouse present a compelling challenge to the widow's capacity for adjustment. The mental health practitioner supporting her in the recovery process is in a key position to prevent and ameliorate the subsequent dysfunction that can occur. This chapter is based on the author's experience as a clinical social worker at Cancer Care, Incorporated, a community-based social agency serving the needs of advanced cancer patients and their families. In this setting, there is opportunity for primary prevention through facilitation of normal and healthy expressions of grief within individual and group bereavement therapy.

Widows in the age range from 18 to 46 years, with children under age 18, represent a high-risk population for intense pathological grief reactions and incidence of mental illness. The objectives of this chapter are to identify the special psychosocial needs of the mother-child relationship during bereavement and to explore the effects of the bereavement process and the role of the therapist.

DEATH FOLLOWING CATASTROPHIC ILLNESS

The literature on bereavement amply touches upon the economic, social, medical, and psychological vulnerabilities of the widow. The disruption of a marriage forces her to undergo changes in all areas of her functioning. She not only loses her role as a wife but may, in losing a young husband, suffer financial hardship and dramatic changes in her life-style. She may be forced to return to the work force or to turn to relatives for economic support. Her mourning usually occurs in a climate overburdened by new responsibilities and affronts to her overtaxed family system. Not only must she learn new problem-solving skills to absorb the responsibilities of her dead spouse, she must also adjust to new roles as a single person and single parent. When death follows the cancer experience, it leaves in its wake a devastation of human and economic resources. Usually, the widow has given of herself fully as devoted care giver to her dying spouse. She is already depleted, when strength is demanded for her grief work and recovery after the death event.

Prior to the death, children experience frequent separations from both parents. Their mother spends long hours away from home accompanying father on treatment visits or at the bedside when he is hospitalized. If father dies at home, children's insecurities may be aroused by changes in home routines, intrusions by the hospice team, changes in babysitters, as well as by their adept reading of and sensitivity to parental fears and uncertainties. Often, they suffer lack of attention or too much attention. When a parent is dying at home, a child's home becomes a hospital setting. The child may be exposed to overwhelming stimuli and may form multiple and fleeting attachments to aides and nurses. Loss of these parental substitutes occur along with the loss of the parent.

A long, debilitating illness may be emotionally weakening, leaving a widow even more defenseless than an unexpected death. When death is inevitable and there is time for anticipatory grief and emotional preparation, it is not a forgone conclusion that the subsequent grief process is shorter or the adjustment easier. Death of a young husband, even if anticipated, is still terrible to contemplate, unacceptable, and often denied as possible, even if predicted. Its prematurity shatters and threatens the illusion we all hold that youth offers immunity to death. It destroys cherished fantasies. Young couples expect to die together in old age after the children are raised and their own parents die. Frequently, when a man in his twenties or thirties dies, his estate is in disarray and there is no life insurance. While a protracted illness can offer time to accept the reality of death, to permit deathbed dialogues, to finish up the business of leave-taking, this does not always occur. Both the patient and his spouse need to deny. To maintain hope, to avoid desolation and despair, to endure painful treatments, to continue fighting for life's precious moments, husband-wife collusion in a denial process is usual. Studies by Gerber et al. (1975) have shown that lengthy chronic illness (lasting six months) results in the surviving spouse suffering poor medical adjustment and more intense grief reactions. Peretz (1970) suggested that a person caring for a dying spouse may not allow himself or herself to experience anticipatory grief because of complete involvement with and need to share precious time with the spouse.

Clayton, Parilla, and Bieri (1980) suggested that instead of giving ample opportunity to help the dying in ways precluding post-

mortem guilt, a long period of anticipation may provide fertile soil
for failure and greater guilt. When dying is slow and arduous, it
places on the care giver deprivations and loss of autonomy and freedom, which for some increase ambivalence, rage, and guilt. To prevent this outcome, effective interventions by the therapist might include assisting the family in locating and financing relief through use
of homemakers, aides, and respite hospitalizations. Support groups
for relatives and spouses of cancer patients provide an atmosphere
where there is permission to vent resentments caused by the demands
placed upon them by the patient. Release of these often-perceived,
unacceptable feelings frees the spouse to enhance the quality of the
time left. The bereavement therapist plays a vital role as witness to
the widow's good care-giving efforts. This is especially important
in critical moments of the widow's self-review. For this reason, it
is especially helpful for the therapist to be personally acquainted with
the deceased and his family before the death.

THE BEREAVEMENT PROCESS

Bereavement is "the state of thought, feeling and activity which
is a consequence of a loss of a loved or valued object" (Peretz 1970,
p. 20). Grief can be defined as an intense emotional suffering set
off by a loss. The seminal writers on grief, Lindemann (1944),
Parkes (1972), and Bowlby (1961), have described bereavement as a
complex process that includes psychological and physiological symptoms manifesting themselves behaviorally, which are antithetical to
the establishment of new relationships and restoration of the survivor's
life. Components of the process are characterized in the literature
as three stages: shock (disbelief), despair (protest), and recovery
(resolution). These stages do not always occur in sequential order,
and they may overlap or recur (Parkes 1972).
A familiar subject among widows in bereavement groups is the
interfering attitudes, reactions, and expectations held by significant
others as they define, comment upon, and hold the widow's progres-
sion of grief against timetables. These reactions compound her pain,
her sense of herself as bad, and her hurt and rejection. As time
progresses and the initial period of numbness wears off, her pain increases. Friends may urge her to inhibit her pain. When she feels
too much is expected, she may withdraw from those who make these
demands. As time passes, friends—especially couples—seem to
disappear. She often feels shunned. To preserve friends' acceptance
and maintain their support, she may inhibit her displays of sadness
or withhold her need to talk of her dead partner. Widows who can
risk other losses vent their rage directly or withdraw from old friends

until anger abates. The widow, in the eyes of her peers, is a tragic, feared symbol. "If it happened to her, it can to me and mine!" The acceptance and support of a community of widows within the bereavement group gives her an invaluable opportunity to deal with the additional hurts when important others fail to comfort. Consequently, it is imperative that the therapist recognize that grief work takes considerable time; that it must be regarded as the mourner's own unique process, conducted without shortcuts or timetables. When this attitude is introjected by the widow, it is extremely helpful in its guilt-relieving, supportive aspects. In order to provide this, the therapist must be aware of the influence of his or her own cultural and socialization process.

Bowlby has discussed some of the important variables that influence the capacity and character of the widow's mourning, including her premorbid adjustment, personality structure, childhood experience with loss, meaning and quality of the marital relationship, presence of additional crisis situations prior to or after the loss, and tendencies toward preexisting pathological relationships of an ambivalent or overly dependent nature (1961).

Studies have supported the relationship between lack of environmental support for mourning and difficult postbereavement adjustment. Maddison and Raphael (1975) found that widows with limited access to emotional support from family and friends suffered deterioration in the year following their loss. Bowlby (1980) documented findings that the widow who has the support of her own mother, or a maternal figure, does better in bereavement. Simos (1977) noted that the lack of social validation to permit expression of emotions following a loss brings the bereaved to a clinician. Clearly, the widow's essential and basic need for nurturance and support, if not provided by her environment, can hinder her recovery. Here, the bereavement therapist and representatives of the bereavement group are available resources.

THE WIDOW'S GRIEF

When a love tie is severed, an emotional and behavioral reaction called grief evolves. The loss of a significant person is one of the most severe forms of psychological stress. The pain of grief is a normal part of life. It is the price we all pay for love, the cost of commitment (Parkes 1972). Mourning, which is the expression of grief, involves the specific psychological task of breaking innumerable emotional ties to the lost loved one and freeing oneself for investment and attachment to the living. "The resistance to relinquishment of that which has been lost, to permit the turning towards the enrichment which life still affords, are the polarities of the mourning process" (Simos 1977). In <u>Mourning and Melancholia</u> Freud wrote that "people never willingly abandon a libidinal position, not even when a substitute is already beckoning to them" (1915, p. 244). Mourning involves the painful, protracted struggle to acknowledge the reality of the loss under strong opposition to abandon the attachment. Over time, the bereaved is compelled by reality to acknowledge the death and slowly decathects or withdraws libidinal investment through a process of remembering and reviewing.

Important relationships create numerous associations and connections that must be severed. Each time a severance occurs because of association with the deceased, there is marked emotional pain. Each milestone, anniversary, and opportunity triggering elation or sadness that had customarily been shared—and can no longer be shared—occasions enormous pain. Bereaved widows have shared with members of their group accounts of the many ways their associations with the dead spouses have taken them by surprise. Some widows have resolved to not listen to music while driving. Modern romantic songs with themes of lost love stir pangs of loneliness to such a degree that driving becomes hazardous. Widows with children find their joy in their children's achievements compromised when a spouse is not there to share it. In telling the group about a child's performance in a school play, one widow stated, "He should be here for our proud moments." Mourning takes considerable time and expense of energy and most of it is done by the widow, alone. For this reason, the work of mourning could be conceived of as long-term in nature.

The widow with children frequently has heard from family and friends how fortunate she is to be blessed by the presence of her children. According to others' perceptions, children give her strength, a reason to go on, a direction for her drifting existence. While some widows do feel lucky and can derive gratification and strength as care givers, others feel differently. The latter are reluctant to express freely and honestly the extent for which they resent their children. Angry feelings provoked by children's demands are socially unacceptable if they are expressed, but they are permitted in bereavement groups. The widow is concerned about the impression she is making and how she ought to be reacting or feeling toward her children. She is grateful for the opportunity to be authentic, yet still be accepted.

The mother's conscious intention to provide what she knows her children need may be eclipsed by her own current feelings of deprivation as well as by suppressed and repressed unmet childhood needs. The small, powerless child she was may rise from the depths of her unconscious, seeking gratification. A recently bereaved widow in individual therapy shared the following thoughts with her therapist: "I feel too much like a deserted, frightened child. I know my daughter's sadness and loneliness is awful, yet I am unable to keep giving.

Her needs are too great and she keeps drawing from me. I see myself in her."

Winnicott (1981) has acknowledged the importance of the quality of the mother's experiences in infancy and childhood in determining the quality of mothering she is able to offer her children. "Her memories of having been cared for either help or hinder her in her own experiences as a mother" (p. 92). In his view, there is a basic assumption that babies are born into a human environment that is either good enough or adaptive. He does not sentimentalize or idealize a mother's devotion to her children. His emphasis is that most mothers are not perfect but are "ordinary devoted mothers" (p. 125). In discussing some of the beneficial effects of mothers' "mended failures," he contributes toward relieving a bereaved mother's guilt. He allows for, and amplifies, the bases that exist for mother's hate, and he suggests that "hate acknowledged leaves room for the enjoyment of the bond that can exist between mother and child." It is important for the therapist to listen for and permit verbalization of a mother's ambivalence. As unacceptable feelings are freely expressed and nonjudgmentally accepted in the presence of a therapist or group, the widow frequently regains her capacity to adapt to her child's needs. When, upon the assessment of her therapist, it appears she cannot regain this adaptive ability quickly enough to avoid deprivation for her children, concrete suggestions can be made. These may include the use of babysitters, surrogates, and extended family. The therapist can help the widow to identify where mending is needed and how to go about it.

An additional task for the therapist is to assist the widow in both developing and actualizing already present self-nurturing skills. These can be drawn from her internalized good objects and good-enough mothering experiences. As she is encouraged to identify, respect, and satisfy her personal needs through mothering herself, often she can become more available to her children. For a time, especially in the absence of external support networks, the therapist may be needed by the widow from within the transference as a parental figure or even as a stand-in for the dead spouse.

THE CHILD'S GRIEF

Loss of an important attachment bond creates considerable disorganization, insecurity, and pain for the child as well as for the adult. The young child's anxiety and rage are usually focused on the surviving parent. The child reacts to death with fear for his or her own safety and may need to know that the surviving parent will remain as a reliable source of vital supplies, protection, care, and abundant love. He or she may fear another abandonment or be angry at the parent's failure or inability to prevent the loss. Acting out and aggressive behavior that provokes punishment may relieve some of the child's guilt but is a further burden to the parent. If the widow is aware of the grief process and can view her child's negative behavior with some objectivity, understanding that it is an attempt at coping with loss, she can endure those reactions more easily.

Controversies still surround the question of whether children and adolescents are capable of responding to a major loss with an authentic mourning response. In exploring reactions to separation and loss in children, Bowlby stressed the persistent demand for the return of the lost love object and the inability to renounce it (1980). These features characterize the nonadaptive reaction to loss in adults. Recent studies of adult patients in psychoanalysis who lost a parent in childhood or adolescence have confirmed that expressions of grief, acceptance of the reality of the loss, and decathexis of the lost parent have not occurred.

Fleming and Altshul (1963) and Wolfenstein (1966) share the impression that children are developmentally unready to do the work of mourning. They continue to deny the finality and reality of the loss and erect defenses against the related affects that prove vulnerable to subsequent confrontations with separation and losses in adulthood. These therapists have taken the position that the capacity to mourn is the byproduct of successful resolution of the developmental tasks worked through in adolescence. This often includes renegotiation of the rapprochement sequence of the separation-individuation process. The psychic structures evolving from resolution of the separation-individuation crisis promote the capacities for self-object differentiation, constancy, reality testing, and tolerance of ambivalence necessary for enduring the painful work of mourning (Edwards 1981). Regardless of children's capacity to mourn, the alliance with the surviving parent and relatives to work therapeutically with them around their grief is invaluable. The bereavement therapist's goal is to support and strengthen these alliances. The mother, to the degree that she has successfully mourned, can lend herself to the child, using the tools received in her own therapy. Specifically, these are a model of listening and communicating and knowledge of grief as a process. For the widow with children, inherent in her therapist's role are facets of both educator and good-enough parent that she can identify with and translate into her own increasingly more beneficial interactions with her child.

Like the adult, the child's handling of grief is deeply influenced by the treatment he or she receives from significant others, primarily the mother. In assessing the specific needs of a child, especially one who is perceived as having emotional difficulties as a result of a major loss, it is important to clarify his premorbid adjustment and to determine the quality of his relationship with his parents. Previous problems are usually exacerbated by bereavement. It is necessary to distinguish to what extent the child is responding to the loss itself and to the strange or different behavior of his widowed parent. A child's response to loss is strongly colored by his stage in ego and cognitive development as well as by the kind of information or misinformation he has received. Important data that help the therapist to understand a child's reactions include how, when, and by whom the information about the death was presented. How the surviving parent wishes and expects her child to respond is another factor that influences the child's response.

THE THERAPEUTIC RELATIONSHIP:
CASE ILLUSTRATION

The case of the A family illustrates the therapist's efforts to ease the pain of grief in a specific mother-child relationship. It is an example that clarifies the interaction between the mourning of a mother and child. It demonstrates their difficulty in renouncing the lost love object and shows their poignant efforts to force the dead father to return through their visible suffering and vindictive rage against each other and the world.

Mrs. A is a 32-year-old mother of two sons: four-year-old Bobby and 20-month-old Jay. She was widowed a year ago when her 40-year-old husband, Fred, a brilliant architect, died of brain cancer after two years of increasing debilitation. Her purpose in seeking help was to arrange for the necessary supportive services so that Fred could die at home. The children had been farmed out to friends and Fred was being nursed by his parents in their home. The couple wanted desperately to share their remaining time together in their own home. Mrs. A regards her success in achieving this goal as her first step toward adulthood. A dependent woman lacking in confidence and self-esteem, in losing her husband she experienced abandonment of a benign, protective parent who also carried a heavy maternal function for the two sons. Despite opportunity for anticipatory grief, her intense despair and depression following the death has lingered.

Mrs. A's gratification in motherhood had always had its limit. After her husband's death, she missed most profoundly her role as a cherished wife and had been able to share her resentment at Fred for leaving her alone. She showed considerable awareness in acknowledging that four-year-old Bobby had become the primary target for her rage. He was a painful reminder of his father, resembling him in both appearance and temperament. Six months after Fred's death, Bobby started to wet the bed, suffered from nightmares, and displayed

increasing hostility toward his baby brother. Mrs. A was concerned
that he had not cried or showed sadness about his father's death and
that he rarely spoke spontaneously about his father. Bobby's sleep
disturbances were conceptualized as reflecting both his anxieties
about his father's death and the disturbances in his relationship with
mother. In children, it is the fear of losing the love object that makes
sleep dangerous for them. Through his disturbances, he effectively
managed to secure the presence and physical contact with mother during the night. It became clear to the therapist and Mrs. A that she
had great difficulty tolerating Bobby's attempts to individuate and de-
tach himself from her.

She was terrified of experiencing other losses of those she loved
and responded with rigid overprotectiveness. Bobby's night fears,
on close investigation, revealed themselves as projections of his aggressive impulses, directed toward both his mother and his sibling
rival (perceived as mother's favorite). With awareness of these dynamics and the support of her therapist, Mrs. A was able to relax
her control and provide Bobby with age-appropriate freedoms and responsibilities. His response was immediate and gratifying. His bed-
wetting lessened and he began to have, as he called them, "sweet, instead of scary dreams."

Despite her perceptiveness and intelligence, Mrs. A felt helpless, resourceless, and angry in coping with her children's demands.
This was identified as her way of convincing Fred that he was needed
and that he must come back. Once this was worked through and her
rage at him expressed and accepted, she was free to direct her energies and take initiative in supplying Bobby and Jay with acceptable
outlets for release of their physical and aggressive impulses, as well
as enriching opportunities for developing social skills.

At one point, Bobby went through a period of running away or
hiding from her in parks and supermarkets. This was particularly
significant and threatening to his mother because of her marked separation anxieties and fears. In view of her intense concern and in
the interest of obtaining an objective assessment of Bobby's needs,
he was seen directly by a therapist for several months. Like his
mother, he proved to be highly intelligent and capable of fine psychological understanding. In sessions of play therapy, his story games
revealed his belief that father was taken away and his thinking that he
could come back, that he was "lost." Since mother made no effort
to "find him," he was angry at her; he was also frightened and in need
of reassurance that if he was lost, he would be found. Feeling rejected, he, too, was angry at father for not returning home. Mrs. A
told him that "God took Daddy to heaven, but no one knows where that
is." He was filled with questions about where heaven is located—in
the sky, in the church? He daydreamed of being a pilot in order "to

see Daddy in the sky." Since his conceptual development limited his comprehension of abstractions, religious imagery used by the family— words like <u>soul</u> and <u>spirit</u>—were open to his embellishments and misconceptions. His preoccupation with death and fears about illness and hospitals were dramatized in his play. This became the subject for direct, honest, realistic discussion in his therapy. The automobile crashes he dramatized, his play acting of dying, ended with his proof of human invincibility. He was also frightened that all he had witnessed could happen to him because adults could not stop it. Themes in his sessions pointed both to his difficulty in conceptualizing the irreversibility of his loss and to distortions caused by Mrs. A's own conflicts, which colored her talks with him about what "<u>dead</u> really means." In their grief both held to the hope that "we'd get Daddy back."

As in this situation, the symptoms of children—especially very young children—often represent their adaptation to a parent's unconscious wishes and emotional conflicts. The therapist's continued flexibility and availability to assist and support both mother and sons in the process of their grief work remain essential if they are to accept this major loss as a real, irreversible, common event in their lives.

Mrs. A has made significant strides in adjusting to her loss. She has used therapeutic support to give up her social withdrawal and has begun to participate in recreational and educational activities. She experiences the time away from her children as renewing and nurturing; she has compiled a roster of competent babysitters and permits allocation for this expense in her budget. She has learned to modify her self-expectations as a single parent and is accepting, with less guilt, the realistic limits of her capacity to give. She perceives herself as a caring, well-intentioned, and "good enough" parent. In becoming therapeutically wise about grief, she has spontaneously recognized subtle indications of grief in her children and has both encouraged and facilitated more direct expression. While these responses to treatment are significant, there is still considerable grief work to be accomplished before she can find restitution for what she has lost.

For the therapist, Mrs. A's loss must be understood in its fullest implications. It must be related to past losses; personality structure; developmental problems of separation-individuation; cultural, religious, social, and family attitudes and models of handling loss; her coping style, ego strengths, and deficits; as well as realistic and available opportunities for restitution and renewal. It is important that the therapist distinguish normal grief from more pathological variants or severe depressions. To this diagnostic challenge are the additional demands present when working with those who suffer varying degrees of depression. At times, help is received with slight appreciation and the benefits are even questioned. On occasion, there is rejection because it fails to meet her needs in restoring what is lost. Widows stuck in the phase of despair (Parkes 1972) are angry and deeply ambivalent. A combination of pleading for help and rejecting it often causes family and friends to be distant or give up on the widow. The therapist can experience this as irritating and wearing but should consider the behavior from an adaptational point of view as one feature of a reparative process that occurs when there is a loss of something vital to psychic structure and integration. Nevertheless, the therapist must struggle to manage uncomfortable countertransference reactions. At times, the therapist may feel depleted, helpless, inadequate, or impotent. All of these responses require awareness if they are not to impair the therapist's capacity to listen, empathize, and make judgments in pacing and selecting interventions.

To be effective, the therapist in bereavement work is required to have more than a solid base of theoretical training in psychodynamic principles of human behavior, mourning, separation-individuation, and crisis management. There must be a continued commitment to broadening awareness of his or her own characteristic defenses in response to attitudes and feelings pertaining to the powerful issues of loss, death, illness, and dependency.

CONCLUSION

As survivors of a death following catastrophic illness, the widow and her children often face serious psychosocial problems of adjustment and a difficult bereavement. The widow's natural mourning response to the loss frequently diminishes her capacity to meet the needs of her children. When she is helped to be aware of her own and her children's needs in the mourning process and is provided with support and validation through bereavement therapy, all family members seem to benefit. The therapist can model and impart to the widow effective attitudes toward death and approaches to communicating feelings of loss that she can use with her children.

REFERENCES

Bowlby, J. 1980. Attachment and Loss, vol. 3. New York: Basic Books.

_____. 1961. "Process of Mourning." International Journal of Psychoanalysis 42: 317-40.

Clayton, P. J., R. H. Parilla, Jr., and M. D. Bieri. 1980. "Methodological Problems in Assessing the Relationship between Acuteness of Death and the Bereavement Outcome." In Psychosocial Aspects of Cardiovascular Disease, edited by J. Reiffel, R. DeBellis, L. C. Mark, A. H. Kutscher, P. R. Patterson, and B. Schoenberg, pp. 267-76. New York: Columbia University Press.

Edwards, J. 1981. Separation-Individuation. New York: Gardner Press.

Fleming, J., and S. Altshul. 1963. "Activation of Mourning and Growth by Psycho-Analysis." International Journal of Psychoanalysis 44: 419-31.

Freud, S. 1915. Mourning and Melancholia. Stan. ed., vol. 14. London: Hogarth Press.

Gerber, I., A. Wiener, D. Battin, and A. M. Arkin. 1975. "Brief Therapy to the Aged Bereaved." In Bereavement: Its Psychosocial Aspects, edited by B. Schoenberg, I. Gerber, A. Wiener, A. H. Kutscher, D. Peretz, and A. C. Carr, pp. 310-33. New York: Columbia University Press.

Lindemann, E. 1944. "Symptomatology and Management of Acute Grief." American Journal of Psychiatry 101: 144-48.

Maddison, D., and B. Raphael. 1975. "Conjugal Bereavement and the Social Network." In Bereavement: Its Psychosocial Aspects, edited by B. Schoenberg, I. Gerber, A. Wiener, A. H. Kutscher, D. Peretz, and A. C. Carr, pp. 26-40. New York: Columbia University Press.

Parkes, C. M. 1972. Bereavement: Studies in Grief in Adult Life. New York: International Universities Press.

Peretz, D. 1970. "Reactions to Loss." In Loss and Grief: Psychological Management in Medical Practice, edited by B. Schoenberg, A. C. Carr, D. Peretz, and A. H. Kutscher, pp. 20-35. New York: Columbia University Press.

Simos, B. 1977. "Grief Therapy to Facilitate Healthy Restitution." Social Casework 58: 331-42.

Winnicott, D. 1981. Boundary and Space. New York: Brunner-Mazel.

Wolfenstein, M. 1966. "How Is Mourning Possible?" In Psychoanalytic Study of the Child, vol. 21, pp. 93-123. New York: International Universities Press.

6

Is There Sex after Death?
Five Widows' Stories

Jacqueline Rose Hott

We do not know what heaven or hell is really like for the person who has died, but we are becoming more aware of the personal sexual heavens and hells, the sexual highs and lows, of a surviving spouse. In order to put sexuality and its role in a survivor's life in perspective, this chapter discusses the specific observations and experiences of five widows and comments on the more general issues of a widow's sexual life. The women—Ann, Lesley, Ruth, Marie, and Jane—are in middle to late adulthood. All physically healthy themselves, they became widowed after eight and one-half to over thirty-five years of marriage.

ANN

Sixty-five years old, Ann has just retired as a laboratory technician.

> My second marriage is easier than my first. My first marriage was not as fulfilling. The second marriage is better, just based on sex alone. My husband had a coronary 12 to 13 years before his death. He died as the result of a massive coronary. I never wanted to strain him in those last years. He would bring me to orgasm manually and I always felt guilty. My contact with the world after his death was limited. Initially, it was just that life went on. I was invited to dinners as a single person. I never thought of myself as a threat to my old friends. They were reciprocating after over 25 years of friendship. I wasn't looking for male companionship, at least not consciously. My sexuality was buried. One of my friends asked me to meet

someone in a similar situation. I met Alex six months later.
We dated and were married in about a year. That was my first
sex since my husband died. Our relationship was more of a
problem in terms of extended family as a problem—not sex.
My fantasy sort of lay buried, but all of life is a trade-off. What
does coming alive mean to me? It means reaching out and being
a whole person, not hiding. Sex is one ingredient of life, a
part of all aspects of functioning.

LESLEY

Lesley is a 59-year-old librarian.

Coming alive—you mean sexually? I never did. I don't know
why. I was 44 and it was just too traumatic. My husband was
sick and impotent for a year before his death. He had returned
home from the hospital to no sex. It was a very hard year. It
was a very traumatic year, including sexually. So successfully
did I bury it that I was scared to ever have it come back. My
daughter said it was so traumatic that I never risked it again.
Maybe she's right, but then there haven't been too many opportunities. Did you know I hallucinated for one year? There was
a prescience there whenever I was awake or asleep. In my
teens, I can only say I was very popular and that later, with
the tentative attempts that men made, I turned them off. Whatever the attraction had been before when I was young, I turned
it off now. My husband was sick for that whole year. After he
died, I hallucinated a whole year. Sex was not with it, so I
went to graduate school to be a librarian. Had I not been happy
there, I think I would have needed therapy. I went into menopause at the same time. I was given Premarin because I had
anxieties, and sexual desires came back when I was on the Premarin. Then my vagina dried up without it. Fantasies stopped.
When I was taking Premarin, I had sexual dreams. It was only
for about three to four months, and I was surprised at the side
effects. My reaction was that this was a cure for being frigid.
Now, I take half a Valium for anxiety.
   My weight gain has been more disturbing to me than anything
else. I sublimated that first year and it didn't revive my sexuality. I think it could be revived. I'm still fond of men. I
find them attractive, and the right man in the right spot would
revive this. I don't know if I dream now. I don't remember the
dreams if I do. Masturbation was an outlet that first year, and
then that need subsided. I never had a feeling that my parents

didn't approve of, but I would like to quote my father. Did you know that he was a doctor? "I'd like to apologize," he would say, "for the entire medical profession." He meant that he knew that no one talked to me at all. I wasn't given one decent piece of advice. I'm making sure that my daughter has no guilt. We all dispensed with our guilt. My daughter is married now. She always had a boyfriend. My son said that she's the one woman whose father died when she was a teenager who wasn't having trouble with men.

One of the nursing faculty spoke to me about hallucinating. The doctor said I was just feeling guilt. But I had no guilt. They said that I was schizophrenic. The first that I heard about hallucinations being normal was when Vietnam war brides in Time magazine were hallucinating. The nurse on the faculty told me, "Hallucinate as long as you need it; then it will go away." And she was right. Now I don't feel anything except sadness, unfinished business. But there is, subconsciously, a buildup that passes like a ripple, and that's what it is when you're getting ready to feel anxious. My mother was very insulting because I didn't remarry. I felt that the children might not like it. Now, in their heads, they're solicitous and good. They'd like to make it up right because they're married and they feel that I should be. It's a different relationship than what would have happened had my husband not died. Our roles are reversed now. My father said that I shouldn't sympathize and I shouldn't be sad, that I should be whatever I wanted to be. My mother said, "You won't meet any men as long as you're a librarian." There are lots of men in the library, but they're not for me.

RUTH

Ruth is a 58-year-old teacher.

Sex—I didn't think about it for a long while. We didn't have sex for at least ten years before my husband's death because we had inadequate birth control. My husband was 13 years older than I. I was 38 when my third daughter, who was unplanned, was born. My husband was going through bankruptcy and this affected his morale. He had respiratory and allergic problems. He was on medication. I just wasn't knowledgeable about what kind of sex life people had. We had a wonderful relationship. I just accepted that, but we never discussed it. It never occurred to me that it was a problem. When I heard about it, I thought that it was too late. Now I've been a widow for seven years. My daughter is away from home at school. I realize the need for touch and kissing, not as much as for sex. By chance, about two years after my husband's death a married man approached me. I was ready. I realized what was open to me. It helped that he was married, because the relationship didn't need commitment. I was thankful for it. I was surprised, excited, very much self-centered in what feelings and sensations there were. I never really admitted that I had a sex drive to my-self. Now there's no reason not to do it. I gave myself permis-sion.

I met a man recently at a singles place, and we've been to-gether ever since—not really living together, but we're at each other's houses. Not permanently, but we do social things to-gether. We travel together, but he doesn't sleep at my home while my daughter is there. I'm just not ready to have her know that. She knows that we go together, but I just don't want her to see us sleeping together. There's a change in my attitude. I have no pregnancy worries now. He's sensual in all the senses, much more than my husband had ever been. There is great joy in our relationship. He hasn't been able to introduce me to his family, though. He's divorced, and he's going through a loss—not only of his wife but of five children. I'm ready to let the world know what change has happened in me.

MARIE

Marie is a 38-year-old nurse.

Sex—there's no sex without love for me. We had a wonderful relationship, had good sexual appetite in marriage, but my libido changed after my husband's death. In our marriage, we had always been physically affectionate and spontaneous. In the hospital, when he had his brain tumor diagnosed, I had a lot of sexual urges because I wanted to deny the whole thing. "If he's able to do this, then there's nothing wrong with him," I thought, but he couldn't have sex because it would increase his inter-cranial pressure. When we came home, he was home for eight months. He apologized that he wasn't a real husband. He tried to pleasure me, and I would feel guilty. It was really meeting his need more than mine. I was very fearful at night, just hold-ing him. The last thing I'd say to him each night was, "I love you," because if he died during the night, I wanted him to know that. And I wanted me to know that I had said it. He looked at me as a lifeline. After he died, it was like everything died. It never entered my consciousness to have sex. Somebody gave me a book about widows. It was awful. It was abhorrent. How could anybody have sex after a husband's death? I felt dead. I wanted to lie down next to him. I really had no choices. I lost my father when I was five months pregnant with my third child. My mother had been married forty-five years at that time, and I cried to her, "I had him for only eight and one-half years; you had your husband for forty-five years." I lost my husband and my best friend. I wanted to scream at people who said, "You're young, you'll make a new life. It's not normal to live like this." I knew what they meant. Why do they allude to sex rather than saying it? Soon after my husband's death, I was approached by a close friend who came to visit me at home. I was appalled, revolted. I actually vomited in the kitchen sink. What sacrilege! After that time, I only went out with couples. I still felt married. I played games with myself, making believe that my husband was home. The next sexual contact—or attempt—was by a colleague of my husband. I laughed at that one. A year and a half later I met Joe, newly divorced, who had had a crush on me years ago. We danced together and the juices started flowing; I felt alive. I was surprised, like flashing lights. I was taken aback that I could feel that way. We've been married since August, and my sexual appetite amazes him. Sometimes I feel guilty, because I recall that I turned my husband away in those early years when we had three kids all under the age of five. We had decided not to have any more children. I think that's part of what I feel sexually.

JANE

Jane is a 40-year-old social worker.

Sexually? I never felt dead. I put up all sorts of walls around myself. My husband died suddenly at age 34. My three children found him dead in the living room from a myocardial infarction. I compartmentalized very well. I could cut a piece off for months: the physical images, the insides coming out. The most important thing to me was the agony of children without a father, making sure of the ongoingness after the loss. I lost a friend, a teddy bear, touch, warmth. I could talk about losing touch; I couldn't talk about losing sex. My friends were outgoing—not just couples, but my close family. My first sexual contact was with a cousin. We had sex; I felt good about it. It's easy to feel that, well, I did it and it's not that bad. I have lots of fantasies to fit in. I was able to separate myself and my goals. I felt confident. I had new perceptions. I was learning about other people. I could enrich myself. By the time I met the man I married, I was ready to enrich a new marriage in openness and sharing and heightening pleasure. I found the relationship that I had had between my first husband and this husband was helped by a second relationship. People can reach out in their own time frame. The issue is not sexuality. Sexuality is just another piece of what they've lost. It connotes too many different things to me—loving intimacy, door closers and openers. Sexuality is too complicated a word. We should use neutral words, like touch, talk, time out, friend, trust, teddy bear. We have to continue to live.

Recent census figures show that over 10 percent of our population, over 20 million people, are over the age of 65. Ten million are over age 75, with only 5 percent living in institutions. Women outnumber men by 3:2 in the over-65 age group. One stress that differentially affects males and females is the loss of a spouse. Since the male's life expectancy is somewhat shorter than the female's and most women tend to marry men older than themselves, there is an ever-increasing number of older widowed women in the older aging group. Many of these women have not been trained to cope by themselves, and this increases their disability. Widows are not homogeneous. Attitudes and life-styles differ greatly according to age, previous marital relationship, health status, educational level, and vocation. Widowhood produces grief and depression, not homogeneity. There is a difference between grief and depression. Grief is an affective sadness, suffered as the result of losing a close personal relationship, and is unassociated with affects of guilt or shame because of repressed hostility toward the lost person. Normal grief is self-limiting and seldom leads to serious impairment of the usual activities, suicidal thoughts, or serious domestic disturbances. Depression has its roots in unconscious guilt arising from interpersonal issues—perhaps from unconscious ambivalence and hostility—with resentful and aggressive impulses directed toward persons who are the objects of an undesired obligation, such as the child whose dependency prevents the mother's remarriage. The hostile impulses, originally directed toward other persons, become directed against the self in depression. Like anxiety, depression is often associated with a decrease in sexual activity and desire. Because physiological changes are associated in later mid-life and in the elderly with a decrease in sexual desire and activity, many health professionals assume that there is a greater decrease in sexual appetite, desire, and gratification than actually occurs. Depression is often a prominent symptom after the loss of a spouse, and concomitant with fatigue, it is the enemy of sexual functioning in women as well as in men.

In addition to being a matter of physiology, sexual functioning is inextricably entwined with one's life situation and place in the life cycle. It is a delicate and mysterious thing for people of all ages. Taking a sex history is essential in order to distinguish between loss of desire and lack of opportunity, between dysfunction because of life stress or dysfunction because of longstanding physiological or emotional problems. The widow's previous patterns of interest and motivation for sexual activity and gratification in marriage (and even before) constitute part of the sex history. Did physical illness, lack of education, genuine apathy about sex, or a long-term dysfunctional relationship in marriage affect her sexual desires and attitudes? Health professionals should offer support for those who continue to be sexually interested and motivated, encouraging their sexual expressions throughout therapy and enabling those who have no wish to express themselves sexually to sublimate those drives in their own way. As always, prevention is better than treatment.

Working with women and men to help them retain sexuality after the loss of a spouse means dealing with and understanding sexual spirits and ghosts that have existed for a lifetime. Sexuality is only one facet of the whole personality. Problems arising in sexual expression result from difficulty in the entire personality. Anxieties and fears that are expressed sexually are not limited to that area. Fear of intercourse can be related to fear of closeness and intimacy. Fear of enjoying sexual relationships can be tied to not feeling worthwhile or not deserving of enjoyment in any area. Fear of loss and abandonment can be linked with general feelings of unlovableness and guilt.

Sex can be used in various ways. Many women use sex as a way to gain security through identification with men who they feel are stronger than themselves, who will protect them, and who apparently have more secure positions. Some women describe the wish for a relationship with a younger man as part of this. Sex can be used as an outlet for anxiety, as a way to get reassurance about lovableness and attractiveness, as a way to gain power and control, and as a way to relieve emotional tension. A woman who may fear getting emotionally involved can get a false feeling of being alive and in love during the sex act. Possession of a man in this way temporarily relieves some women's feelings of emptiness, boredom, and weakness. Others may use sex to prove their independence and their willingness to take risks. They have many affairs, although basically they are contemptuous and prudish. There are women who avoid sex because they feel it subjugates, lowers, and exposes them.

What is healthy sex? A healthy use of sex is to fulfill physically a close emotional relationship, to increase closeness, to allow great self-revelation to the loved partner. It is constructive and satisfying and a mutual enterprise that is part of the whole relationship, not the end-all and be-all of existence. Sex, as a part of the whole relationship, helps healthy development of the entire person.

It is important to give widows permission to be sexual, to use whatever kinds of sexual activities feel good. Sexual activity covers a wide spectrum. The opportunity to explore the broad emotional aspects of sexuality should be offered. Options should be explored and direction given toward choosing the one that fits best. These options include communal living, homosexuality, extramarital relationships, and sharing a lover. The focus should be less on dysfunction and more on so-called healthy reactions to sexuality that allow for responsible freedom and responsible relationships. Trust and acceptance should be encouraged. Each of us has an urge to grow. With help, self-confidence can be fostered so that the widow will develop a more realistic attitude toward life in general and toward love and sex in particular

7

The Art of Living
with Change

Brenda Lukeman

What do we have that we can lose?

The experience of loss is an experience that we all dread, one which we go through continually on many levels. Most of our life consists of preventing loss, holding on to what we have and to the image of self that is our personal identity. There is a strange paradox here, because the more we hold on, the more insecure we can feel, the less able to endure the change that must inevitably come.

In order to safeguard against deep loss, against the feeling of being left empty and alone, we spend a great deal of time accumulating many things and then holding on to them. We accumulate money, friends, skills, academic degrees. Then we become very proud of our possessions. Temporarily, we may feel full and overflowing, but then we become afraid of losing what we have gained. This cycle repeats itself continuously.

Because of the fear of loss, we become driven to do more, to have more, to prevent ourselves from being empty. We want to feel constantly that we are becoming bigger and better, wiser and wiser. Our sense of ourselves wants to expand.

However, along with the process of accumulation, the process of attachment appears. Attachment is painful. It restricts us and is motivated by a sense of desperation and fear. It becomes exacerbated by a deeper sense that loss is inevitable and that some day we may be alone.

Why do we attach and cling so tenaciously? Attachment arises out of misunderstanding about who we truly are. We become identified with our possessions and accumulations. When they change or are taken away, we feel as if we have lost a part of ourselves, as if somehow we have become smaller. For many, there is a sense of personal failure here. Each loss has somehow diminished the self.

The very process of change itself is experienced frequently as loss. As change is inevitable, and even necessary, many individuals are constantly experiencing loss.

Women, in particular, undergo change continuously, if only on a physical basis. During the process of maturation, menstruation, pregnancy, childbearing, nursing, and menopause, many changes occur—both physically and emotionally. For some women the sense of identity is intimately connected to their childbearing function. During all of these periods of change, women feel particularly vulnerable and often experience a lack of stability. They are undergoing changes and fluctuations in their sense of identity. They are not exactly sure of who they are.

After the birth of a child, not only do some women experience joy, but they also encounter a real period of grieving, of loss. They may be experiencing the physical loss of the baby from within their body, or of the pregnancy period. They have lost their identity as a pregnant woman and there may be difficulty making the transition to the role of new mother. There may be a time of grieving for the loss of oneself as a young, carefree woman.

When any loss occurs for a woman (whether of a body part, relationship, and so forth), there is a strong tendency to internalize and take on some blame for what has happened. Loss is usually experienced as bad. We may feel that we have done something wrong or that we had to endure the loss because somehow we were not good enough. Some women feel as though they are being punished. These unconscious factors have a strong influence. There is a loss of self-esteem.

All sense of loss is ultimately the loss of self-esteem. Even when a loved one is lost, we feel personally reduced and diminished. Our sense of identity is threatened and shaken by each loss we undergo.

We know who we are in a relationship. When the relationship is gone, our sense of ourselves goes with it, too. We wonder what went wrong and why we are no longer lovable.

When a part of the body is maimed, diseased, or lost, many women experience a significant change in identity. Many individuals identify themselves with their bodies and with the images they present. This is the external sense of identity, knowing ourselves as we appear in another's eyes. When our external image changes or when people react differently to us, we feel that we are no longer the same person. When part of the body becomes ill or has undergone significant change, the sense of our value and beauty becomes shaken and diminished.

Feelings of loss and grieving occur because we feel that we are not lovable, beautiful, or valuable anymore. Most grieving is grieving for ourselves. It may be grieving for a part of our lives or for some aspiration that we have held on to, which will not be realized now. Even after we have lost someone we loved, we may feel unconsciously that this person has abandoned us because we were not good enough, not really lovable.

After each experience of loss, a period of self-evaluation and even mourning takes place. There is a need for time for renewal and repair. The period of mourning is a period of withdrawal, which takes place so that we can become whole again. The questions we deal with at this time are What is my function? How can I see myself as worthy both in my own eyes and in the eyes of another? Loss and failure are intertwined: "Now that I have lost something, I feel as though I have failed. How can I regain my footing?" What we really are doing is examining our sense of identity.

The basic question being addressed is the question, "Who am I?" If I have lost a breast, a baby, or a loved one, then who am I now? How will others respond to me? This question must be addressed and brought out into the open. Is there another sense of identity I can attain that will not be subject to fluctuation and loss? What is there about me that will never go away? In order to aid an individual who is experiencing grief and loss, one must encourage a new sense of identity, a new way of experiencing and knowing the self.

Depression often follows grieving and loss because we feel that we are not important anymore; some people feel that they have become nothing. The question reappears: Who am I really? There is an expanding and a diminishing sense of identity. When we identify ourselves with that which is transient and can be lost in a moment, then inevitably fear, insecurity, loss, and depression must follow. When we find another source of self, we are protected from this buffeting. Is there some way we can see who we are beyond all of the physical changes? Another strong source of the depression that accompanies loss is the sense of futility and meaninglessness that many experience. What is the point of living and struggling if everything that is gained will be taken away? This is the unspoken question that haunts us.

Now it is necessary to reevaluate the nature of change itself. Is all change loss? Rather than seeing change as loss, rather than experiencing it as personal failure, we can learn to see change as fundamental and nourishing to all life. We can learn to see it as a significant prelude to growth and newness.

Nothing stays the same. When we stop resisting change, we become a part of the larger universe, part of the endless flow. After we do this, there is a small leap to be made so that we begin to see that, basically, there is nothing that we can lose, just as there is nothing we can ever hold on to. Whatever we have experienced or attained is now a part of ourselves forever. We cannot hold it and we cannot let it go. It is just a part of our larger nature. Everything is always in a state of flux. When we see this deeply, then we can become joyful and trusting in all circumstances, knowing that change is only the constant and gracious movement of life.

Part II
Miscarriage, Perinatal Death, and Abortion

8

Women's Grief Reactions following Spontaneous Abortion

Phyllis C. Leppert

Women experience a definite, intense grief reaction following the death of an embryo in early first trimester abortion. This reaction is characteristic of all grief reactions but is of shorter duration. The pattern of grief is identical to that following the loss of an infant or young child and includes the following stages: (1) shock, (2) disorganization, (3) volatile emotions, (4) guilt, (5) loss and loneliness, (6) relief, and (7) reestablishment. Since women often need the most help in the stage of guilt, they should be given ample time to discuss their feelings, to cry, and to initiate the grief process.

That the grief process exists is not unexpected, as it has been well documented that an affectionate bond is initiated to the fetus by the pregnant woman very early in gestation. This occurs universally in married and unmarried women and is handled in different ways by them as individuals. In wanted pregnancies the woman has begun to project her dreams for the unborn baby into the future and develops an attachment to the fetus. This happens at a time when most of her social circle does not know that she is pregnant and when the father of the baby has not had time to develop a feeling for the baby. Thus, if the pregnancy is lost, the woman feels isolated in her grief. This disassociation of the grief between husband and wife often leads to misunderstandings and marital stress. In counseling sessions conducted in a private practice setting, the intensity of emotions demonstrated by the mothers is strong, regardless of the gestational age. However, the fathers display some emotional distance in early gestation and are more concerned for their wives' welfare.

Counseling sessions are initiated at the time of the initial diagnosis of spontaneous abortion and immediately following the physical stability of the woman who miscarried. The woman and her spouse or partner are told that it is quite common to feel anger, bitterness, or sadness and that these are acceptable emotions that can be discussed. The importance of communication between the parents is also stressed. This initial statement is followed by a 30- to 45-minute interview in which the mother and the baby's father are allowed to express their feelings and concerns. Telephone follow-up contact is maintained in the weeks that follow. The number of times this contact is made is determined by each couple's need or by concern on the part of the practice staff. A physical examination is conducted four to six weeks after the spontaneous abortion, and this is followed by a final supportive counseling session.

The shock of the loss of a pregnancy and its affectionate bond with the fetus is followed by sobs and tears. Occasionally, the shock of the realization is denied or rationalized. Some women look back on their pregnancy and state that they knew it was "not right from the beginning." Some express a "why me?" feeling. One husband told his wife that he felt suddenly vulnerable and developed a sense of inability to control the events in his life. In some way, all couples feel that they are uncomfortable around friends and relatives who do not appear to understand their grief. They are often urged to forget the miscarriage and get on with life but find this philosophy difficult to accept.

Guilt is difficult for these women. This stage of grief takes the longest to work through, and it is the stage at which the couple needs the most support. Some women think they had a spontaneous abortion because they jogged or forgot to eat properly. Others have to deal with real etiological factors such as heavy smoking or exposure to anesthetics. Many couples find that participation in an epidemiological study investigating the cause of spontaneous abortion helps them to understand why the miscarriage occurred, thus easing their guilt.

All women reach the last stages of grief approximately three to four months following the spontaneous abortion. They are now prepared to consider another pregnancy.

BIBLIOGRAPHY

Kavanaugh, R. 1974. Facing Death. Baltimore: Penguin Books.

Kennall, J. H., et al. 1970. "The Mourning Response of Parents to the Death of a Newborn Infant." New England Journal of Medicine 283: 344.

Peppers, L. G., and R. J. Knapp. 1980. Motherhood and Mourning. New York: Praeger.

Seitz, P., and L. Warrich. 1974. "Perinatal Death: The Grieving Mother." American Journal of Nursing 74:2028.

Wolff, J. R., et al. "The Emotional Reaction to Stillbirth." American Journal of Obstetrics and Gynecology 108: 73-77.

Zahourek, R., and J. Jensen. 1973. "Grieving and the Loss of a Newborn." American Journal of Nursing 73:836.

9

The Incomplete Pregnancy

Susan F. Leslie

In one year, I had a stillbirth followed eight months later by a miscarriage. When the stillbirth happened, I was nine months pregnant and five days past my due date. The pregnancy had been wonderful, and I enjoyed every minute of it. There was never morning sickness, and my checkups had been routine with no problems. It was a textbook pregnancy, the happiest nine months of my life.

From day one, we had so much fun planning for that baby—choosing names, guessing the sex, painting the nursery, picking out clothes, and telling my two sisters and six brothers that they would become aunts and uncles for the first time. My husband and I went to every single childbirth class and practiced breathing every night.

On Saturday morning, December 19, 1981, we drove up to Larchmont to buy a Christmas tree. I mentioned to Tom that the baby wasn't moving and it concerned me a bit. In the car I felt as if something were leaking from me, as if, maybe, my water had broken. We stopped at Tom's brother's house, and I ran into the bathroom to find a greenish-brown substance was leaking from me. (I was later to learn that this was meconium—almost always signifying that the baby is in fetal distress or dead.) I called my doctor, and she told me to go right to the hospital and straight to the maternity ward. She sounded calm, but I was terrified.

As we walked out of the elevator, four people approached us immediately and asked, "Are you the Leslies?" They whisked us into the labor room and put a fetal monitor on me. I knew this red carpet treatment was anything but routine. I looked over at Tommy and realized that he had no idea that anything could be wrong. I knew what they were going to tell me. I remember thinking how nice it would be for him if they could delay the bad news for awhile longer. I knew he was ready and anxious to be a father.

The nurse and a staff doctor put a few fetal monitors on me. They thought one didn't work, so they went and got another one. There was no heartbeat. I kept asking, "What's the matter? Can't you get a heartbeat?" No one would answer me. The staff doctor finally said, "Dr. Carter will be here in a few minutes." It made me angry that he would say nothing more, that he must be saving the dirty work for Dr. Carter. A few minutes later, she walked into the room looking sad and shaking her head. She said, "I'm really sorry." I asked, "Is the baby dead?" She answered, "Yes."

My response was odd. I said only, "Oh really" (as if someone had told me it was raining outside). I might have been in shock or maybe I was just numb. Tommy started crying and then I started crying. We were hugging each other. Dr. Carter said, "I'll leave you alone for a minute." I felt terribly confused and started to question what I possibly could have done wrong. I had eaten all the right foods and had taken good care of myself. I never had any alcohol or coffee. I just could not figure it out.

A little later, Dr. Carter walked in and said, "We have to make a decision. We are not sure why the baby died, but there is a possibility now that you could be in some danger." She carefully explained that if the reason was not cord complications, there was a high risk of my hemorrhaging when they took the baby. The next step was to take a blood sample for laboratory analysis. It later turned out that the test results were inconclusive, so a hematologist was put on call to deal with the possible emergency of placenta previa. Dr. Carter also explained that they had to induce labor with Pitocin and since the baby was not alive to help the labor, it could be a long labor. I wanted to know why they could not perform a C-section and just get it over with. They were not sure of my clotting factors and surgery would be too risky. Also, Dr. Carter had to think of future pregnancies, and she felt that 16 hours of labor, although horrible now, was the right decision in order to have normal deliveries in the future. In retrospect, I am glad that this decision was made.

Labor was induced and became violent quite rapidly. They also gave me a considerable amount of Demerol, which made me feel confused. Tommy sat on my right side, holding my hand. He was crying and telling me how much he loved me. I kept asking him why he was crying. (I was later to find out that he was worried about losing me.) His crying frightened me. I told him to call his father because it seemed as if he needed someone and no one was helping him at the hospital. He finally did call, and his father came to the hospital.

The whole thing was a confusing nightmare. I was frightened at knowing that there was a dead baby in my womb. I wanted to escape the feeling of death that overcame me. I told Dr. Carter that I wanted to be "knocked out" in the delivery room. She agreed to do this when

I was ten centimeters dilated. The labor nurses were patient even though I was in pain and kept asking for more medication.

As the labor was progressing, one nurse walked in and said, "Look, Tom. You can see the baby's head and all the blonde hair." When she walked out, I said, "Tommy, is that a new nurse? Doesn't she know the baby is dead?" He answered, "No, it's the same nurse who has been here all night." I was angry at her comment. Not until months later was I able to come to the conflicting opinion that I felt great warmth toward that nurse. She was one of the few people who acknowledged that our baby was a person, whether dead or alive, and that it should be treated that way.

When the baby was delivered and I was in recovery with Tommy, that same nurse came in and told us our little girl was beautiful and that we should see her. Under the influence of drugs, I decided not to see the baby. I thought it would be too painful. That was a decision I have regretted. Tommy did go to see the baby. He said she was pretty and she looked just like me. Of course, that made me feel more as if a part of me had died. I spent the next four months asking him every day what she looked like. He told me the same thing over and over again, but I just couldn't hear it enough. I wanted to hear every detail. To this day, I still like to hear what she looked like. I love the nurse for convincing him to see that baby.

I also regret that no one ever really tried to explain to me why it would be good to see the baby. I think if I had been asked a second time when the drugs wore off, I would have said, "Yes."

There was a sense of relief when I woke up in the recovery room. I remember thinking, "It's finally over." But it didn't take long before I was to realize that the physical pain was nothing compared with the mental pain that followed. Dr. Carter told us that the baby was a beautiful, healthy-looking girl, perfectly formed, but with cord complications. The doctor cried with us.

My doctor went through all sorts of red tape to insist that we be put in a private room. It happened to be next to the nursery. Although I felt sad when I heard babies crying, I don't feel that there was anything wrong with being in that room. She understood the importance of our being together and alone. They could not get a cot for Tom. He sat on a chair and wouldn't let go of me. He kept telling me how much he loved me and how happy he was that I was all right. It was Sunday morning, around 6 A.M. We fell asleep for awhile until they brought in breakfast. Neither of us could eat. I am happy that he was allowed to stay with me. I needed him there. I kept holding my stomach and felt so empty without the baby there.

Most of the nurses were wonderful and accommodating. They came in and introduced themselves. Each one told me how sorry she was that our baby had died and how upset all of the maternity floor staff was. They also told me that everyone kept saying how beautiful the baby was. I felt proud that my baby was beautiful, yet horrified that such an innocent little baby had to die the way she did. I hoped it wasn't painful for her.

At no time during my pregnancy had I been prepared for the grief I had to face when my baby died. In childbirth classes the subject never came up.

Tommy's father and his stepmother had been at the hospital almost the whole night while I was in labor. They were supportive to Tom but for some reason, which is unclear to me, had told the other children not to call us, that we wanted to be left alone for a few days. This decision (made without consulting us) turned out to be quite a painful one. My family called me and some even came into the hospital to see me right away. My father (whom I hadn't spoken to in three years) called me at the hospital. The first 24 hours is such a crucial time. It is necessary to talk and to have someone who will listen. It was painful that no one in Tommy's family called when we needed them the most. When they finally did call, there were excuses such as, "We were told you wanted to be left alone," or "I didn't know what to say." I had finally told Tom to call them. I thought it would make it easier for him. His sister, Barbara, called because she realized that she was protecting her own feelings, and she knew we would need her. She turned out to be a lifeline for us over the next year, listening to everything and making it clear that she was always available. Tom's mother had died of cancer not long before our baby died. Barbara told us, "Mother would have wanted to help you two through this tragedy, but you can be sure that she is up in heaven giving God some 'hell' for causing this to happen!" A few laughs later we all agreed that this was true. Then Barbara gave me two beautiful antique pins that were her mother's and said, "I know mother would like you to have these." I was touched by this gesture and will never forget it. The pins will always remind me of my baby girl who died.

Twenty-four hours after delivery, Dr. Carter released me from the hospital. She said it was doing me no good to be there, and I wasn't sleeping. This was the longest period in my life that I had gone without sleep. I was exhausted but couldn't fall asleep. My mind wouldn't stop thinking of the past two days.

The cab ride home from the hospital with no baby was painful. During my whole pregnancy, I had thought often of leaving the hospital with our new baby as the first step into the new role of becoming parents. For months, I imagined that day. We even planned to have my youngest brother take movies with our camera so we could one day show the little baby how it left the hospital to enter the world. When I got into that cab with no baby, I felt empty. The pain when the cab hit each pothole on the way home was excruciating because of my episiotomy, but it was mild compared with my heartache.

When I arrived home, I discovered that all of my baby things were gone. The room was empty. A few people in Tommy's family had made the decision that I should not come home to see baby things around. There is a possibility that in the confusion I was a part of that decision. They had driven down before I returned home, but no one stayed long enough to see us. I felt violated. Other people were deciding what was to be done about my life and my affairs. No one asked what I wanted or what would make me feel better. I searched around for my baby books. Everything had been removed. There was no trace of anything even remotely connected with my baby. What I wanted to see was gone. It made me feel like a child. I kept asking Tommy where by baby things were. I worried that they would not be taken care of properly. I was told that they had been wrapped in tissue and boxed. I don't know why I was so concerned. Maybe it was because these things were all that was left to hold on to that were a part of my baby. I couldn't relax until I went to my sister-in-law's house. We walked down to her basement to find all of my stuff piled up, uncovered, in a dusty corner. I couldn't wait to take everything home to be put in a safe, clean place.

I remember something else that had bothered me: Dr. Carter wanted me to take tranquilizers. Although I wasn't sleeping, I didn't want to sleep. I'm not sure why. I remember telling her emphatically that I would not take tranquilizers. What bothered me was, why only for me? Why weren't tranquilizers prescribed for Tommy too? Couldn't he be as upset? No one recognized or acknowledged this. He was a nonperson, who happened to be married to me. No one acknowledged that his baby had also died. In my mind, the only major difference between us was the physcial pain I had suffered. In many ways, my physical pain was easier than the emotional trauma he felt until the delivery was over and he was sure I was out of danger.

The only support that we received in the hospital was from Dr. Carter. There was no one else there for us—no social worker, nurse, priest, or anyone who could help in our confusion. We needed to talk and we needed someone to listen. With the exception of one or two people, we had no one who would listen during this time. The few people who called us had plenty to say but not much time to listen. We heard comments such as, "This was the doctor's fault," "Well, you just have to try again," and "At least you never knew the baby." Clearly, people did not know what to say. I suppose they thought we would feel better if they played down the tragedy, but this made us feel worse and more alone.

I felt isolated. I could not communicate my feelings to other people. No one seemed to want to listen, they didn't understand. They tried to cheer me up and get my mind off the baby, but there was nothing else I wanted to talk about. I needed to talk. I wanted to feel the pain. I wanted to cry. I didn't want people diverting my attention from my baby.

I couldn't understand the intense feeling of loss that overcame me. I couldn't get the image of the labor room and the hospital room out of my mind. I couldn't fall asleep at night, and I cried every night.

My crying wasn't limited only to night. Most days I would sit on the couch crying, reading, and watching television. I had no concept of time. Tom usually walked in the door when he got home from work to find me crying. Then we would often cry together. I guess it was the first time during the day that he had time to cry. I am thankful that he is such a wonderful and understanding man. He let me grieve as much as I wanted or needed, and we spent hours talking about the tragedy and how it was affecting our lives. We have always communicated well, and this helped us cope better.

I did not want to go out, but Tommy convinced me that it was time to go shopping together a week after returning from the hospital. I was still in maternity clothes, since my body had not returned to normal yet. Strangers asked me, "When is the baby due?" I felt guilty about still looking pregnant. If there had been a health baby at home, I could have said, "I just had a baby." Instead, I'd say, "I just lost a baby." I ran home and cried the rest of the day. This was the last time I wore maternity clothes. One of my friends took me to buy some baggy sweatsuit pants, which happened to be stylish then. They were the only things that fit me, and I wore them every day for months.

The tension was mostly released by my crying. I guess I was lucky to be able to cry so easily, but I'll never forget an incident that was uncharacteristic of me. Tommy had gotten tickets for a tennis tournament in Madison Square Garden. It was the end of January and the temperature was about 5°. Before the matches, we were meeting a friend for dinner at a restaurant. Tommy had gotten the name of the restaurant wrong, and we walked around Madison Square Garden three times looking for it. Finally, I couldn't take the cold any longer and started to scream at the top of my lungs, "How could you be so stupid!" I continued to scream as I realized that no one was around and no one could hear me. It felt good to scream on that freezing cold night. Then I started to cry. We had never before had a fight or even raised our voices at each other. It scared me. When I apologized to Tom, I was in agony. How could I have yelled at the person I love most in this world? He understood and helped ease the guilt I felt. He was comforting and understanding, yet I wondered how much more stress he could take. It seemed that he was always the stronger one.

For months, my mother called me every day. I'll never forget that. I started to depend on her calls. I guess she was grieving that her first grandchild had died. I also think it confused her because she had had nine healthy children with no trouble. For her, having babies was easy, too easy.

I can't help being disappointed in some of my friends. Some of my best friends became strangers. Dealing with death was too hard for them. Some avoided calling me for months with excuses such as, "I was told that you wanted to be left alone." They were so uncomfortable on the phone that they couldn't wait to hang up.

One of my oldest friends never called. Eleven months later when his father died, I called him. He listened with disbelief when I told him I thought he didn't like me anymore. To this day I am sure he is confused about my saying this. One social acquaintance called and said, "I'm sorry to hear about your little problem." I wondered what bigger problem I might have ever had.

There were friends, though, who did call often. I was very touched when one of my college roommates called me from Egypt as soon as she received my letter about the baby. Friends whom I hadn't heard from in years called. I needed every bit of support I could get. However, I did become a sounding board for horror stories. People felt they had to tell me stories that were worse than mine. They must have felt that these stories would minimize my loss. It didn't work but only made me feel worse. I finally learned to stop people from doing this. I couldn't bear to see violence on television or even hear about it.

I love the people who let me mourn. They told me how awful it was for my baby to have died. It was a help when someone acknowledged this. I missed that little baby and any opportunity to talk about her was a relief. Sometimes, I was angry at her for dying. Why couldn't she have been stronger?

We made many telephone calls in an attempt to contact support groups. Our attempts were in vain. We were recommended to a psychologist who was supposedly a specialist in this field. The final session with her came two months after my baby died. I told her I was too upset and unable to return to work. I am a flight attendant, and I was not ready to go back to a job where I would be forced to leave my husband and stay in hotel rooms. She told me, "This grief stuff is bullshit" and that she thought I was really upset about going back to a job where all the girls are "skinny and beautiful." I remember asking, "How would you know? You never have experienced the death of a baby." I was disturbed that she could not understand my dilemma but amused that she must not have been on an airplane lately! And this was a person I was paying to help me? I told her I would not need her anymore. This turned out to be one of my better decisions. Immediately I started to feel a little better.

The cycles I went through were crazy. There was no sense to them at all. I would feel good for a week and be out doing things and having fun. Then just the slightest comment, a television commercial, or a phone call could trigger a devastating reaction from me. I was crying and depressed again for the rest of the day. I would have a few bad days, then a good day. I continued on this kind of roller coaster for about four months. For the first time in my life I had no control, and it was frightening. I did notice that, as time went on, the bad days became less frequent. I started to socialize a little, but it was painful. People would see me and say nothing about our baby dying. There was a conspiracy of silence that put a wall between us. It made me angry that no one could tell me they were sorry. For the first time in my life, people were uneasy around me. I didn't know what to do. People walked the other way when they saw me coming. I could tell that they couldn't bear to face me. People would ask Tommy, "How is Susie doing?" I never heard about anyone asking him how he was doing. Once again, no one would acknowledge the fact that Tom was also mourning his baby.

Slowly, things started to get better. We felt that we were finally coping.

After about five months, I was ready to become pregnant again, and the doctor approved. Much to our surprise I conceived that first month. We were relieved not to have the pressure of contrived sex over our heads. Our sex life had been hard as it was. If you are not ready to get pregnant, you are afraid of sex since even with birth control there is a risk of pregnancy. Making love was scary because it reminded me of my failure to carry my baby to delivery safely. I couldn't bear the thought of having another child die inside me.

Tommy and I decided not to tell anyone until I was three months pregnant. I was not ready to hear congratulations; I felt they would be appropriate only when we had a healthy baby. Also, we were constantly getting messages from the outside world that we would be socially acceptable again when we did have a healthy baby. People will be more relieved than we will be, if that is possible. Maybe that is because we will never forget our first baby girl, nor do we want to forget her. That pregnancy was one of the most wonderful times in my life. But the rest of the world wants us to forget it. How do you relay the message that you will never forget, that you don't want to forget?

No one was happier than Dr. Carter that I was pregnant. We had a long talk about what we would do differently this time. The last month would have been the only real difference. I asked her about my baby girl. I think I needed her reassurance that I had done everything I could to have a healthy baby. When I asked her, "Is there anything I should do differently? Was the baby healthy?" she told me not to do anything differently. Then she said, "I hope this doesn't make you feel badly, but I will never forget that baby. That baby was beautiful!" As she spoke, she had tears in her eyes. I love her for saying what she did. It gives me a warm feeling to have another person in this world remember my baby. It's the type of warmth that helps ease the pain. No one else was able to express that warmth to me. I guess it is natural to feel close to one of the few people who saw my baby.

My second pregnancy seemed to be routine until my three-month checkup. We had told people I was pregnant two days before. Since I had the first appointment of the day, Dr. Carter had not arrived yet. Two nurses did the routine tests before she arrived. Then they decided to try to get a heartbeat with the doptone. The first nurse could hear nothing. The two nurses and the receptionist frantically tried every doptone in the office and then told me that the batteries probably needed recharging because they could hear no heartbeat. Dr. Carter walked in and said, "I hear these rookies couldn't get a heartbeat. Let me try." I remember saying, "I've been through this before." As I suspected, she also could hear no heartbeat. I started to cry, and they rushed me over for a sonogram. I became very angry when the sonogram doctor, who knew nothing of my past history, said, "I'm sorry, but it's better that it happened this way." He also gave me no information but said that Dr. Carter would talk to me. I was to learn from her that I had a defective ovum and would need to have a D&C. She made arrangements to put me into the hospital that day.

Once again, Tommy was burdened with the task of relaying bad news. His family must have learned from the first time around, because almost everyone showed up at the hospital before my operation. I was very grateful for their support. It did scare me that I was so calm, almost as if I had expected this to happen. For two weeks after the miscarriage I remember telling people that I was not discouraged. I was determined not to be excluded from the rest of the world again. Yet my first few days home from the hospital were terrible. Tommy was very upset. He kept asking, "What more will you have to go through to have a baby?" At this point, I tried to comfort him and tell him that the physical pain was minor compared with his mental pain. I could see how much he was suffering and felt I had to be strong for him. It was a reversal of the roles we had assumed at the time of the stillbirth.

The first phone calls did not come until three days later—along with the excuses that we had become experts at predicting. One of my biggest concerns was the inability to communicate to friends and family how much we needed their understanding. We had lost enough, but it made us feel worse that they would avoid us again because of this tragedy.

Around the time of my two-week checkup, I started to crash. We reverted back to missing our baby girl. A real and significant part of our lives had died. I guess the second time around I thought I was prepared for what I was going to face. I was wrong.

I lost my concentration. I had difficulty focusing for any period of time on anything. When people spoke to me, I did not hear what they said. The insomnia returned, and I never felt rested.

I lost my appetite and interest in everything. I did not want to leave the apartment. Going to the grocery store around the corner became a major effort. I did not want to see anyone. I had no desire to talk to anyone on the phone, so I didn't answer it. I lost all track of days and time. If my husband was ten minutes late, I started to worry. A choking kind of anxiety overtook my whole body. My breathing became weird. Tom was sensitive to the fact that I felt terrible anxiety about his being late. I would tell myself that it was crazy to be so worried, but my body would not listen. I stood by the window, almost terrorized, until I saw Tom walking up the hill to the apartment.

As soon as the date for my return to work approached, I became panic stricken. I was convinced that my first flight would crash. I wasn't ready to die, and I knew Tommy would fall apart over losing me and being alone. Living my life was like watching a television set. I saw this person (myself) go through the motions of daily life, yet it was all mechanical. I felt numb and detached. Nothing seemed to have a purpose.

Dr. Carter told me that it was not uncommon to feel this way after going through terrible trauma. She referred me to a therapist who, she felt, could help me. It turned out to be a positive relationship. When someone can explain what is happening to you, it can make more sense somehow.

My husband and I have learned to appreciate everything we have.

In retrospect, I can say that much of the pain we experienced was intensified by the lack of support from family, friends, and the hospital. Had this part of our experience been different, we might have been equipped to deal with the tragedy a bit better. Also, I have learned that people really do not know how you feel from an experience like this unless they have been through it themselves.

10

Perinatal Grief as a Disorder of Change: Interventions to Aid Parental Adjustment

Brenda C. Sumrall,
John C. Morrison,
and Sue M. Palmer

Although much work has been done in the field of neonatal and infant loss and subsequent bereavement counseling with the parents and family, little effort has been devoted to stillbirths, spontaneous abortion, and ectopic pregnancies, all of which represent perinatal losses. It is our proposal that the population of patients at risk for these losses be dealt with in a preventive method through team intervention during pregnancy.

Infant and neonatal death rates continue to fall in the United States, as does the number of stillbirths. Yearly statistics reveal a diminution in the country as a whole as well as in the state of Mississippi. Within the authors' own institution, the death rates for neonates have fallen particularly rapidly owing to an obstetric and pediatric team approach to risk identification and intensive patient management. The incidence of fetal deaths, on the other hand, has not fallen nearly as rapidly. In addition, the incidence of spontaneous abortion remains at approximately 15 percent of all pregnancies, while the risk of ectopic pregnancy has risen slightly but not to a significant extent. Therefore, according to the national statistics from 1981, a perinatal loss will strike one pregnancy in seven.

Previously, the early losses such as spontaneous abortions or ectopics were not thought to be correlates of grief and bereavement. Even a stillbirth, because "the baby was not born alive," was not thought to be as traumatic to the family as the neonatal or infant death. Now substantial evidence points toward this not being true. It has been our most recent focus within the perinatal unit to deal with fetal deaths, and we are just beginning (at the University of Mississippi) to deal with grief counseling after spontaneous abortions and ectopic pregnancies.

A good illustrative case of a patient and her family who might be at high risk for perinatal losses is represented by involuntary infertility. Patients who have involuntary infertility are known to be at an increased risk for first and second trimester spontaneous abortions and miscarriages. If the involuntary infertility is the result of tubal problems and/or intrauterine factors, the patient would be at risk for first trimester abortions (12-24 weeks), as well as for ectopic pregnancy (which usually occurs within the first 16 weeks of pregnancy) and for a premature delivery (which would occur prior to the 37th week).

In addition, many maternal disease processes such as sickle cell anemia and diabetes give rise to women at risk for perinatal losses.

Although it is important to understand the frequency and statistical significance of perinatal loss to women, it is even more important to understand the significance of a particular perinatal loss to an individual woman. Pregnancy and birth are two of the most significant events in the life of a woman, and a loss during pregnancy and birth can have a far-reaching impact on the woman and her family. The failure to adjust optimally to this loss can lead to long-lasting emotional disorders, marital disruption and divorce, family dysfunction, sexual difficulties, and a failure to bond with and effectively parent future children.

It is a commonly held misconception that loss during the perinatal period is not as significant as the loss of an older child or a spouse. However, women who have experienced a perinatal loss indicate that it can be difficult to resolve and that it does have a significant effect on the long-term well-being of the woman.

Traditionally, the psychosocial needs of women experiencing prenatal loss have been virtually ignored by the health care provider. When health care providers were aware of the significance of the loss to the women involved, treatment has traditionally been offered in the form of crisis intervention. It usually involved referral at or after the time of loss to a social worker, psychologist, chaplain, or other helping person, who is usually unknown to the woman until the time of the referral.

Crisis intervention as a helping technique is concerned with a rather brief period of adjustment that must follow a crisis. Theory states that an individual suffers pain when there is an unexpected loss of known patterns of coping and while the individual seeks new life patterns. Whether or not this new life pattern is satisfactory depends essentially on how well the individual is able to resolve the change-created problems during the period that follows the crisis. Crisis intervention theory recognizes that although crisis disturbances are brief, adequate or inadequate adjustment to them has far-reaching effects in the life of an individual. Techniques employed in crisis intervention have involved intensive support of the individual and have attempted to maximize the individual's strengths. The helping individual may also find it necessary to intervene with various social systems that may be preventing the bereaved woman from making an optimal adjustment.

Our suggested interventions for women who experience perinatal loss stem from the basis of crisis intervention but also consider the problem as a disorder of change, a change that in many cases can be predicted and for which specific interventions can begin as a preventive measure before the actual crisis occurs. A crisis of change, as defined by David Kaplan (1982), is a brief personal struggle to adapt to changes in both psychological and social areas. Interventions in a disorder of change must be addressed to both psychological and social situations. Women experience change in the form of the predictable transition of pregnancy and birth, but when it is accompanied by unexpected transition into the bereaved state because of losing the pregnancy, a situation develops for which they are usually unprepared and for which they have few coping skills.

Even the women who make maladaptive responses to change are not necessarily mentally ill. In general they do not require psychiatric attention, but rather, their poor coping results from the behavior of others within their social system, the rapidity of changes in their lives, a lack of information, or a lack of decision-making skills.

The individual's attempt to resolve a crisis of change can essentially be described as a problem-solving struggle. The outcome of the struggle is linked to resolving certain coping tasks. The problem solving involves cognitive, affective, and decision-making elements. The decisions made by the individual and their appropriateness allow us to evaluate how adequately the individual is able to cope with her crisis. The goal of intervention, then, is to help the individual to replace her perhaps ineffective problem-solving method with learned, effective ones in order to achieve a good outcome.

Coping with the possibility of perinatal loss involves (1) the cognitive element of understanding and facing the possibility of loss, (2) the affective element of experiencing and voicing emotions and sadness, and (3) making the sometimes difficult decisions associated with one's own health care.

It is our recommendation that all team members involved in caring for the potential high risk patient be involved in education during pregnancy. Information learned about her own situation and potential for loss will serve the woman well in mastering the cognitive portion of coping. The team approach is also necessary in learning affective coping. All members of the health care team should encourage the woman to express feelings about her pregnancy, about the information she is learning, and about any fears she may have concerning the possibility of loss. Early involvement of the woman in decisions relating to her health care can provide valuable experience that will lead to more effective decision making during the crisis. An increased understanding by the woman of the elements involved in health care and decision making by professionals can serve as a valuable guide when the woman herself must make decisions relating to loss.

The social systems involving the woman should be evaluated early in the pregnancy, so that areas of potential problems can be dealt with prior to the crisis. Possible levels of intervention include dealing with family reactions; development of a support group of peers; or intervention with the system of hospital, clinic, or community to modify policy or provide for special needs of the patient.

It should be emphasized that although these recommendations are psychosocial in origin, they apply to each member of the health care team. The multidisciplinary nature of this intervention is one of its greatest strengths. A multidisciplinary intervention creates a "community of concern" with the interventions of each health care professional reinforcing the others in a way that is not possible when any one team member is solely responsible for the emotional well-being of the patient. It is recommended that the same team follow through with involvement during the crisis, if it should in fact occur. When it is inevitable that health care givers outside the original team will become involved during the crisis, they should be introduced into the system of health care as early as possible in the patient's course.

Although the high risk patient is the one who will benefit the most from this type of team intervention, it should be emphasized that 15 percent of all normal pregnancies end in spontaneous abortion and that there are other losses that cannot always be predicted. Therefore, providing team-oriented support and care to all obstetrical patients is desirable.

It is hoped that when these recommendations are followed, the potentially high risk patient will have mastered techniques for understanding her medical problem, that she will feel free to express and face her feelings related to the problem, and that she will be able to make appropriate decisions supported by a concerned health care team. Through this preventive method, it is hoped that maladjustment to perinatal loss and grief can be minimized and that an optimal outcome for the woman can be achieved.

REFERENCE

Kaplan, D. M. 1982. "Interventions for Disorders of Change." Social Work 27:404-10.

BIBLIOGRAPHY

Borg, S. , and J. Lasker. 1981. When Pregnancy Fails. Boston:
  Beacon Press.

Parkes, C. M. 1972. Bereavement: Studies of Grief in Adult Life.
  New York: International Universities Press.

Perlman, H. H. 1957. Social Casework: A Problem-Solving Process.
  Chicago: University of Chicago Press.

Rapoport, L. 1961. "The Concept of Prevention in Social Work."
  Social Work 6:3-12.

Speck, W. , and J. H. Kennell. 1980. "Management of Perinatal
  Death." Pediatrics in Review 2:59-62.

11
The Perinatal Bereavement Team: Development and Functions

Kathleen Leask Capitulo
and
Anthony J. Maffia

Perinatal loss, whether through miscarriage, stillbirth, or neonatal death, was long thought to be a nonevent by lay people and health care professionals alike. Interest in the subject of death and dying and the process of parent-infant bonding by Klaus and Kennell identified perinatal loss as a significant, multifaceted life crisis (Klaus and Kennell 1976).

Although some health providers acknowledge this special loss, few recognize the vast numbers of clients affected annually. In 1980 the New York City Department of Health reported a total of 1,719 infant deaths up to one year of age (1,202 of which were under 28 days of life) and a total of 5,692 fetal deaths (2,771 of which were greater than 13 weeks gestation) (New York City 1980). These statistics validate the need for intervention in all institutions that provide obstetrics and perinatal services.

At Booth Memorial Medical Center in Flushing, New York, the special needs of parents experiencing perinatal loss have been addressed through the formation of a perinatal bereavement team. The team is comprised of highly skilled professionals who are specialists in the area of perinatal bereavement. The three primary team members are the clinical nurse specialist for obstetrics and gynecology, the social worker for obstetrics and gynecology, and a chaplain trained in thanatology.

The need for a formal program was identified by the director of obstetrics and gynecology, who encouraged and supported the team in initiating a hospitalwide program. At the program's inception, a consulting committee was established. It was composed of the director of obstetrics and gynecology; a pediatrician; a psychiatrist; nurses from labor and delivery, postpartum, and the newborn nursery; and the morgue attendant. The consulting committee assisted not only in the development of the program, but also in the education of the staff and, ultimately, in the general acceptance of the philosophy of a bereavement protocol. Following the writing of procedures, the perinatal bereavement program and team were presented to and accepted by the hospital's medical board and became part of Booth's official policy.

The purpose of the team is to provide crisis intervention, support systems, assistance with the grieving process, a therapeutic milieu, and counseling to families who experience stillbirth, fetal demise, neonatal death, second or third trimester pregnancy loss, or the birth of a sick or anomalous child. Referrals of first trimester pregnancy losses from hospital staff and sudden infant death syndrome cases from the emergency department are also accepted.

In addition to counseling families, the team functions as a support system and educational catalyst for professionals in obstetrics and perinatology. Education involved presenting on-unit workshops to all nursing personnel on every shift, speaking at joint medical conferences, and continually inservicing all new personnel on the policies of the program. For this reason the team members attempt to be available for consultation on a 24-hour basis. In the beginning, even if the delivery was at 2:00 A.M., it was essential to serve as a role model and to be present. However, with education of and acceptance by the nursing staff, night calls are less common and the staff is competent to provide appropriate, therapeutic communication and intervention.

When the diagnosis of a fetal problem is suspected or made, a member of the team (usually the nurse) is called by the nursing staff for consultation. The team responds, speaks with the mother and significant others, and assesses the need for intervention. The nurse on the team will stay with the mother during any diagnostic tests and, when possible, for the actual delivery. The baby's father or mother's support person is also encouraged to be present at the delivery. A couple needs to be together during this crisis. The baby's father frequently will stay, when supported by hospital personnel, even when the child is known to be stillborn. The presence of a support person allows the mother to share her grief and increases the cooperation the staff receives from the visitors. One father who witnessed the birth of his stillborn daughter recalled the birth, saying, "I saw her come out with the cord around her neck twice, and then I understood why she died." For him, her death was real.

Heavily medicating the mother for the delivery of a stillborn is not recommended. Mothers who were asleep during the delivery report that they do not believe their babies were born dead and postulate that something may have been done to kill their babies. A mother who is asleep cannot witness the birth. As Peppers and Knapp have pointed out, "A mother who is not allowed to see her baby (after delivery) develops feelings of anger and resentment toward those who have denied her the privilege" (1980, pp. 70-71). Although it may seem cruel for a mother to be awake during this sad birth, it enhances her acceptance of the death and, ultimately, the resolution of her grief.

In speaking with these parents, it is important to acknowledge and validate the loss of their child. Simple statements such as, "I'm sorry, I understand your baby has died" or "I'm sorry" are appropriate and therapeutic. Phrases such as, "You're young, you can have another one," "Forget it, it was a bad dream," or "It's best your baby died, it may have had a problem" have no place in therapeutic communication with the bereaved. While they may serve to ease anxiety on the part of the professional, they literally translate into "I don't care" to the grieving parents (Peppers and Knapp 1980). After the loss of a child, parents frequently blame themselves for the death. Mothers feel a special guilt, having nurtured and borne the baby. A mother may feel that because she worked or missed one vitamin she caused the infant to die. As a general rule, all blame should be dispelled from parents. There is no need to question parents concerning recent sexual activity or missed physician's appointments, as this only perpetuates guilt that will follow the couple for the rest of their lives.

Following the death of their child, parents must make several decisions and are given a variety of options, the first of which is whether or not they wish to see their baby. Parents have the right to see, hold, and touch their child, immediately after the delivery and/or at a later time, if they so desire (O'Donahue 1979). In the delivery room, the infant should be wrapped in a warm baby blanket, held by the nurse, and described to the couple. Positive aspects of the baby's appearance should be emphasized. In cases where there are changes in color or skin (maceration) or congenital defects, the delivery room nurse should explain this to the parents. The mother and father or support person should then be allowed to see and hold the infant, if they wish to do so. Showing the baby in a positive, caring manner has been found to assist the family in acceptance of the death and grief.

The mother should choose whether or not she wants to remain on the maternity floor following delivery. The decision must not be made by her doctor, spouse, family, or nurse. Some women are more comfortable on the obstetrical unit and feel they are being rejected if they are sent off the unit without being consulted. Others, however, do not want to deal with other mothers or newborns at this time. Both feelings should be respected.

Some parents may not desire to see the stillborn at delivery. This may be due to fear that the child is grossly abnormal, desire to forget the event, or inability to cope with the situation at the moment. No one should be forced to view their baby. However, it is found that families frequently do request to see the child at a later time. Therefore, arrangements must be available for the bereaved to see the baby after it has gone to the morgue. The goal of such a viewing is to provide a positive remembrance of the child. Under no circumstances should a baby be shown in the morgue.

At Booth Memorial Medical Center, when a viewing or wake is requested, the baby is dressed in baby clothes and blankets by the morgue attendant or team nurse and is taken to the chapel or chaplain's office. Any pleasant room or office could be used. The mother and/or family is accompanied to the room by the social worker or the mother's nurse. Parents are encouraged to bring clothes for the child, as this enhances the baby's appearance and allows them to give something to their offspring. Strategic placement of clothes, a hat, and blanket markedly improves even a less-than-perfect infant's appearance.

Frequently, the family may wish to hold and examine the baby, particularly the hands, feet, and genitalia. They should be allowed as much time as they desire to say goodbye. In addition, photographs have been found to be therapeutic and should be permitted. At Booth, an instant camera is available for this purpose. A standard hospital photo release form is obtained before pictures are taken. Some parents have returned months later seeking pictures. A copy of the baby's picture is kept in the bereavement file for this reason (O'Donahue 1979).

After a death, people frequently seek support from their religious beliefs. Involvement of the ecumenical team chaplain and clergy of the parent's faith assists the family greatly. Generally, families are encouraged to meet their own needs by exercising all religious rites desired; any type of religious ritual may be practiced within the law. Wakes and funeral services are held in the hospital chapel. This allows the mother to participate during her hospitalization with a maximum number of professional and family support persons. When a mother is confined to her bed for medical reasons, the baby is taken to her room if she requests it.

In several cases families have had elaborate funerals attended by over 30 family members and friends. During these services the baby is often blessed and named, reinforcing the identification of the deceased as a real person. One Hindu father washed his stillborn son in rosewater and dressed him in preparation for cremation.

Burial options are discussed with parents. The team describes private, municipal, and Saint Vincent de Paul arrangements for Roman Catholics (a small plot with a monument). These options are also covered in a pamphlet, "Grieving for Your Baby," which parents receive. Having a written reference enhances their understanding during

this highly stressful period. Parents should be given sufficient time
to reflect on the options, and they should be supported in the decision
they reach. Autopsy consents are explained, emphasizing that an
autopsy is optional and may or may not reveal the cause of death. If
an autopsy is to be performed, it is best to have the wake prior to it.
A viewing may be arranged after the autopsy examination, but it is
less desirable.

Prior to the mother's discharge she is given all available information regarding her baby, including height, weight, footprints, and
a dedication name certificate. These serve as cherished memories.
Parents are prepared for dealing with family, friends, and other children when they return home. Counseling is performed on the normal
physiological and emotional feelings of grief.

Intervention does not end when the couple leaves the hospital.
The team's telephone number is given to the couple, should they have
any questions or just want to talk. During the next week a team member will call them to assess their ability to cope and communicate at
home. In about eight weeks the couple is invited back for a follow-up
interview. At this time the couple meets with the team, autopsy results are given and explained, and parents are given the opportunity
to express their feelings about the loss. Marital, communication,
and sexual problems are identified by the team and appropriate referrals are made, when necessary.

It is often important to emphasize that grief work is important
and necessary (Nessel 1978). Parents may feel they are going crazy,
when the feelings they are experiencing are entirely normal. The
couple should be advised that they will never forget their child and
that from time to time their feelings of loss will be exacerbated.
This is clearly illustrated by Peppers and Knapp's concept of shadow
grief. This type of grief manifests itself on special anniversaries,
birthdays, deathdays, holidays, and the like. On these days people
may appear outwardly happy, but inwardly they mourn the dead infant
(Peppers and Knapp 1980). Where pathological grief reactions are
seen, referrals are made for psychological counseling.

Development of a successful interdisciplinary team is based
upon a unique interplay from several disciplines. Each specialty
brings its own expertise, and together they blend into a therapeutic
support system for clients, professionals, and each other. It is essential that team members be comfortable with their own practice in
order to work both independently and interdependently. Territoriality
has no place in teamwork and can, in fact, cause the end of a well-
intentioned program. Roles will and should overlap. As the team
becomes more experienced and more flexible, roles become more
fluid and open.

Dealing with death, particularly that of a neonate, can be physically and emotionally difficult. Team members should support each

other and foster open communication. After each stillbirth, wake, funeral, or follow-up, time must be made for team members to discuss their own feelings as well as to assess the team's functioning. Periodic conferences with the consulting committee also assist the team in its ongoing work. Although working with families during the crisis of perinatal loss is not easy, it is rewarding. Clients do appreciate the caring, supportive atmosphere generated by the bereavement team. This truly humanistic concern for the bereaved has been demonstrated to be worth the time, effort, and expertise invested. At Booth Memorial it is considered to be a responsibility to assist these special families at a time of special need.

REFERENCES

Klaus, M., and J. Kennell. 1976. Maternal-Infant Bonding. St. Louis: C. V. Mosby.

Nessel, L. 1978. "Support for Parents of Acutely Ill Newborns." Social Work Journal, January, p. 13.

New York City. 1980. Department of Health, Bureau of Vital Statistics.

O'Donahue, N. 1979. "Facilitating the Grief." Journal of Nurse Midwifery 24: 10.

Peppers, L., and R. Knapp. 1980. Motherhood and Mourning. New York: Praeger.

12

Witnessing Loss: Perspective of a Nurse-Clinician

Constance Weiskopf
and
Mahlon S. Hale

The obstetrical service at the John Dempsey Hospital of the University of Connecticut Health Center has become a high risk regional center for the state of Connecticut, joining the high risk neonatal intensive care unit (NNICU) at the hospital. Owing to the high risk population, attending obstetrical physicians, house staff, and nursing staffs have had to readjust their perspective from dealing with a healthy population to caring for a population whose means of entry is a previously identified threat to the health of either the mother or fetus. These issues of change have been witnessed by the psychiatric consultation service, which has increasingly been asked to intervene in patient management and in attendant staff problems. One example of the depth of involvement has been the maintenance of an ongoing support group over the past three years for the NNICU nurses. It has been facilitated by the nurse-clinician on the psychiatric consultation team and structured in such a way that opportunities to participate are available for all nursing shifts. For all the professionals involved in care on this high risk unit, however, a common concern has emerged: how to deal with the constant threat of loss, which is no longer measured in percentages from an otherwise healthy clientele, as each case runs the risk of having a graver outcome than the precedent cohort.

John Bowlby (1969) has said that "loss of a loved person is one of the most intensely powerful experiences any human being can suffer." He added that the pain of witnessing such loss is at least as intense an experience because onlookers often feel so impotent to help. In this chapter we relate Bowlby's comments, through case examples, to some of the critical issues of loss. It is, of course, at the interface of the highly skilled and the supremely needy that all of us come to grips with the ironies of the limits of our personal effectiveness.

Bowlby (1969) has noted the dearth of empirical data documenting individual age-related responses to losses of different kinds and under differing circumstances. In our review of the literature, it is curious that we were unable to find references to guide us in our analysis of the case examples. We know that other health care units have had similar experiences, but documentation of reactions of care givers to specific losses is hard to find.

Peretz (1970) has commented on the effects of loss and death to physicians and nurses and their identification of themselves as helping persons. The cases presented in this chapter exemplify the challenge that physicians and nurses believe they must address. They also represent a threat in that they hold the potential to undo otherwise strongly internalized beliefs unless they are addressed by helpers for the helpers.

CASE 1

The patient, a 27-year-old mother of three young girls, worked full-time at a local insurance company. She was admitted to the high risk service at 26 weeks of pregnancy with the diagnosis of placenta previa. Her husband left the family home the night of her admission. While he kept in close contact with his wife and the staff during the admission, we have never worked out the degree to which his abandonment may have affected the course. Both husband and wife were Jehovah's Witnesses. The patient remained in the hospital for one week and then was discharged, but she began to bleed and returned to the hospital for the duration of her pregnancy. As a result, she became one of the first long-term patients on the obstetrical unit.

Initially, the nursing staff viewed this woman as an extremely strong person, which may have been partially because of their knowledge of the husband's abandonment. While the medical focus was consistently concerned over the possible loss of the fetus, this condition remained stable and they often reverted to social concerns. These were verbalized by observations such as, she "lacks support." They felt that they became one of her major support systems. Unfortunately, this attitude was to eventually severely complicate their relationship with and management of the patient. The patient was, in fact, quite competent and engaging, and the staff rapidly shared (we learned retrospectively) much about what was happening elsewhere on the unit and much about their personal lives with her. Two examples of the staff's overextension—perhaps so labeled retrospectively—were their decisions to throw a baby shower for the patient and to invite her to a staff party at a nearby restaurant. These activities were sanctioned by the medical staff. Late on the night of the party, the patient began to bleed and began to contract. It is important to note that prior to these events the patient had signed the standard form to refuse any blood transfusions.

The next morning a male infant was delivered by C-section. In the process of closure the patient began to bleed. Volume expanders were given and both the patient's mother and husband were frantically contacted, as was the hospital lawyer. However, they refused to allow blood transfusions and the patient died. The mother remained stoic and said, "It was Jehovah's will." The husband, while emotionally wrought, also said he had made the right decision. This was the first maternal loss the staff had experienced on this obstetrics unit.

The psychiatric consultation service was contacted that day for an emergency staff meeting. The nurse-clinician was met by a room full of nurses from the obstetrics, labor and delivery, intensive care, and neonatal services. The staff was inconsolable. Members were angry, tearful, depressed, and resentful, with much anger displaced upon the mother and the husband. Some staff reenacted the chain of events, seemingly to undo them. They reported that the physicians were equally upset. One attending obstetrician has since refused to treat another Jehovah's Witness as a patient.

It appeared to the psychiatric consultants that the entire staff was totally unprepared to deal with this outcome, as the loss was unanticipated, or—if you will—denied. Overinvolved, strongly attached, perhaps allowing the length of confinement to allay their anxiety, they were not prepared for the worst outcome scenario. The loss was sudden, quite traumatic, and permanent. In their eyes, the loss could have been avoided. In subsequent group meetings, staff members began to raise a most significant "what if" issue, namely, what would occur if staff became so involved with every admission. As the second case will illustrate, this very real concern was rapidly processed by the group, for in the next month they had a similar case.

CASE 2

A 24-year-old unwed Polish émigré who worked for a charitable organization was admitted at 25 weeks of pregnancy to the high risk obstetrics unit. She had a single ventricle with pulmonary stenosis and had been advised to terminate her pregnancy. She had refused, ostensibly out of strong religious beliefs. She was to remain at bed rest until her delivery and was felt to have a fifty-fifty chance of survival. There had been very few documented cases with her anomaly, so the staff was uncertain how to treat her. A detailed history was taken and the father was found to be a Polish-speaking refugee without legal papers. His commitment to this woman seemed highly questionable.

Within the first week of admission, the staff called a psychiatric consultation, a social service consultation, and a meeting with the hospital chaplain. Dialogues about patient issues were frequently and openly held between staff and the consultants. As the due date approached, a meeting was arranged between the staffs of the obstetrics neonatal intensive care unit and the adult intensive care unit to address possible issues about her care and the care of the baby. The issue of potential loss of either mother or baby was addressed openly. Staff members also made references to the precedent case. The medical and nursing staffs seemed assured that they had done all they could to anticipate and meet this patient's medical, emotional, and social needs. Our ongoing dialogue with the patient led us to believe that she concurred totally with the staffs' plans for her and her infant. She told us that she looked forward to C-section. She was concerned that she might die, but she felt that she had addressed the issue with her family and the staff and felt optimistic. A special team was identified by staff to be called in at any time to deliver her, including cardiologists, obstetricians, and nurses. A C-section was called on a weekend, and the team responded as had been planned. A healthy baby boy was delivered and the mother survived.

From follow-up visits with the patient and from subsequent staff groups as well, we learned that moving toward some very painful issues of anticipatory loss required much effort on the part of all involved. However, this process prepared both patient and staff for undesirable as well as optimal outcomes, and it appeared to give them a sense of control that was lacking in the previous case. The staff had felt initial relief because the care of the patient had been shared. This also facilitated their maintaining boundaries with the patient. The patient benefited because her needs had been addressed in an open atmosphere that permitted both understanding of the complex nature of the problems she faced and recruitment of multiple resources to deal with them.

It did appear to us with this case that each member of the team and each team section had clear definitions of role and an understanding of the contribution others might make. On the other hand, one can hypothesize that the intense involvement with the first case was so painful that the staff took measures to alter those forces that would lead to their greater—perhaps pathologic—involvement.

It is our hope that these illustrations have provided some insight into the direction that care givers' responses to loss can take and how these responses may be altered to protect both staff and patient when they overreach professional boundaries. While we hesitate to generalize, we believe that the present atmosphere on this obstetrics unit, where we continue to facilitate biweekly meetings, is substantially different from the atmosphere at the time during which the first case arose. By assisting care givers to recognize and deal with their own anticipation of a reaction to loss as well as the reactions of patients and their families, we believe a healthy balance between compassion, sensitivity, and professionalism may be established for optimal care giving.

REFERENCES

Bowlby, J. 1969. Attachment and Loss. New York: Basic Books.

Peretz, D. 1970. "Reactions to Loss." In Loss and Grief: Psychological Management in Medical Practice, edited by B. Schoenberg, A. C. Carr, D. Peretz, and A. H. Kutscher, pp. 20-35. New York: Columbia University Press.

BIBLIOGRAPHY

Brim, O. G., H. E. Freeman, S. Levine, and N. A. Scotch, eds. 1970. The Dying Patient. New York: Russell Sage Foundation.

Grossman, S., and J. Strain. 1975. Psychological Care of the Medically Ill. New York: Appleton-Century-Crofts.

13

Personal Loss in Ectopic Pregnancy

David L. Rosenfeld

Conception in humans occurs in the ampulla of the fallopian
tube. On the third day after fertilization, the zygote will enter the
endometrial cavity of the uterus, and by the sixth gestational day it
will begin inplanting within the endometrial layer. When there is a
disruption of this normal reproductive process, which results in extrauterine or ectopic implantation, the pregnancy will fail and a gynecologic emergency will result.

Ectopic pregnancies are unique to humans, with aberrant implantation occurring very rarely in subhuman primates. Even with
experimental arrest of a fertilized ovum within the oviduct of an in-
fraprimate, eccyesis will seldom result (Thibault 1972). Ninety-
nine percent of ectopic implantations are within the fallopian tube.

The incidence of ectopic pregnancy has been increasing world-
wide and varies with the socioeconomic composition of the population
(Curran 1980; Kitchen et al. 1979). One in forty to one in three hundred of all pregnancies are extrauterine. The number of ectopic
pregnancies has tripled in the United States from 1967 to 1977. This
increase has paralleled the increase in sexually transmitted diseases
(Curran 1980).

Ectopic pregnancy may result from situations that retard the
passage of the embryo into the endometrial cavity, conditions that increase tubal receptivity to implantation, or factors intrinsic in the
conceptus itself (Bronson 1977). Evidence of prior tubal infection,
or chronic salpingitis, has been identified in 15 to 40 percent of women
at the time of surgery for ectopic pregnancy (Sherman et al. 1982).
Recent estimates suggest that between 500,000 and one million women
in the United States will suffer from acute salpingitis or its sequelae
yearly. Approximately 20 percent of patients known to have acute
salpingitis are subsequently infertile (Curran 1980; Westrum 1980).

In a Swedish study, 5 percent of 412 women studied prospectively for more than six years after laparoscopically verified diagnoses of pelvic inflammatory disease developed ectopic pregnancies, a more than fourfold increase in risk over a nonaffected population (Westrum 1980).

The majority of women with ectopic pregnancies do not have evidence of salpingitis. Congenital anomalies of the fallopian tube are quite rare and endometriosis of the tubal mucosa is infrequent. Abnormalities in tubal anatomy have been noted in the women exposed in utero to diethylstilbestrol (DES), and this has resulted in an increase in the rate of ectopic pregnancy (from 1 to 5 percent) in this group of patients (Rosenfeld and Bronson 1980). There is also an increase in the risk of tubal pregnancy (10 to 20 percent) in women following tubal surgery for infertility.

There appears to be an association between the use of the intrauterine device (IUD) and an increase in the risk of ectopic pregnancy (Kitchen et al. 1979; Malhotra and Chaudhwy 1982). While an IUD will reduce the risk of intrauterine pregnancy by 99.5 percent, the occurrence of tubal pregnancy is reduced only by 95 percent. The risk of ectopic pregnancy in IUD wearers increases with the duration of use and with the use of medicated devices. There is also a higher-than-normal incidence of tubal pregnancy in women conceiving after removal of an IUD. Postcoital contraception with high dose estrogen preparations or contraception with low dose progestins, both of which will retard tubal transport, increase the risk of tubal implantation.

A retrospective survey of 83 patients with tubal ectopic pregnancy in a Canadian population with a low incidence of chronic salpingitis showed a statistically significant association between prior spontaneous abortion and subsequent ectopic pregnancy. The author suggested that this might result from ovulatory dysfunction with delayed ovulation and fertilization of an overripe ovum (Honore 1979). Nevertheless, ectopic pregnancies have no higher frequency of chromosomal abnormalities than in utero conceptuses of comparable embryonic ages (Elias et al. 1981).

The cost of an ectopic pregnancy is high in terms of maternal mortality and compromised fertility. Ectopic pregnancies account for 6 to 15 percent of all maternal deaths in the United States (Bronson 1977; Kitchen et al. 1979). Following an ectopic pregnancy, 30 to 70 percent of women will be infertile, and 6 to 27 percent will have a second ectopic pregnancy if conception does occur (Franklin, Zeiderman, and Laemmle 1973; Kitchen et al. 1979; Schenker, Eyal, and Polishuk 1972; Sherman et al. 1982). Moreover, 20 to 30 percent of women with ectopic pregnancies have a prior history of infertility (Sherman et al. 1982). Postectopic pregnancy infertility is higher in women over age 30, in women who had never been pregnant prior to the ectopic gestation, in women with coexistent tubal disease, and in instances where the pregnancy results in tubal rupture.

The use of sensitive radioimmunoassays for the detection and quantitation of human chorionic gonadotrophin (HCG), earlier diagnosis with the use of pelvic sonography, and the prompt and liberal use of diagnostic laparoscopy have all contributed to a significant drop in the number of ruptured ectopic pregnancies (Breen 1970; Kadar, Devare, and Romero 1981; Kitchen et al. 1979; Lundstrom et al. 1979; Schwartz and DiPietro 1980). Earlier detection has significantly contributed to the reduction in maternal mortality and morbidity as a result of ectopic gestation and has resulted in improvements in the subsequent pregnancy rate in these women. In 1970 Breen noted that 80 percent of ectopic pregnancies were ruptured at the time of diagnosis, with treatment consisting primarily of tubal salpingectomy (1970). In 1982 Sherman et al., using modern biomedical techniques, reported that 58 percent of ectopic pregnancies were diagnosed intact (1982). With the use of microsurgical techniques, an unruptured ectopic pregnancy can be treated conservatively with preservation of the involved tube. The procedure will not increase the operative morbidity or the risk of subsequent ectopic pregnancy in these patients. Moreover, recent data confirm an improvement in the live birthrate in these individuals (DeCherney, Maheaux, and Naftolin 1982; Kitchen et al. 1979; Langer et al. 1982; Sherman et al. 1982).

The occurrence of an ectopic pregnancy has a profound effect on the couple. An ectopic pregnancy requires hospitalization and emergency surgery, a frightening experience for the couple. The individual's grief is compounded by the pain and prolonged recovery that result from the operative procedure. A scar remains to forever remind the woman of her failure.

In addition to disappointment at the unsuccessful termination of the pregnancy, there is a mourning process following the ectopic pregnancy. Even in the early stages of pregnancy, the fetus has become a person in the minds of the couple. A period of shock, suffering, and recovery may be seen after the death of a beloved object, albeit one that is potential and anonymous. This mourning process is similar to that which is seen in the loss of wish fulfillment. Moreover, guilt, shame, embarrassment, and feelings of inadequacy and personal defectiveness may accompany the mourning process (Berger 1977).

These individuals feel guilt and self-blame, wondering if their action might have caused such a catastrophe. Myths about the prevention of miscarriage are common in many societies (Borg and Lasker 1981). There is a sense of depression fueled by an internalized anger. The question "Why me?" is often asked. Many women feel they are being punished for past actions.

The couple's grief is compounded by their belief that a failed pregnancy is viewed by society as sexual dysfunction, with fertility associated with female genital success and male potency. The woman suffers from her concern that she is depriving her husband of a family. Their inability to have a successful pregnancy violates the biblical doctrine to be fruitful and multiply—the cardinal principle of marriage. Childlessness signifies dysfunction and disorganization in one's attempt to fulfill the vital function of the family, that of replacement. As a defense mechanism, these couples will often isolate themselves from social contacts with family and friends.

In addition to feeling socially unworthy and inadequate, these women suffer from injury to their self-esteem, self-image, and sexuality. They develop feelings of bodily defectiveness and a loss of sexual attractiveness, especially when the fallopian tube has been removed or the other tube is found to be damaged. Sexual function may be impaired by the stresses imposed by trying to conceive, the ordeal of breeding versus that of lovemaking, or the fear of another abnormal pregnancy. There is great anxiety over the subsequent birth of a defective child because of this defective pregnancy. Moreover, these couples are most frightened about the occurrence of another ectopic pregnancy with its potential risks, surgery, possible castration, and repeated failure. For these reasons, counseling services may help the couples to reduce anxiety and to rework the concepts of sexuality, self-image, and self-esteem, thereby helping them cope with their loss and prepare for the future (Rosenfeld and Mitchell 1979).

REFERENCES

Berger, D. N. 1977. "The Role of the Psychiatrist in a Reproductive Biology Clinic." Fertility and Sterility 28:141.

Borg, S., and J. Lasker. 1981. When Pregnancy Fails. Boston: Beacon Press.

Breen, J. 1970. "A 21 Year Survey of 654 Ectopic Pregnancies." American Journal of Obstetrics and Gynecology 106:1004.

Bronson, R. A. 1977. "Tubal Pregnancy and Infertility." Fertility and Sterility 28:221.

Curran, J. W. 1980. "Economic Consequences of Pelvic Inflammatory Disease in the United States." American Journal of Obstetrics and Gynecology 138:848.

DeCherney, A. H., R. Maheaux, and F. Naftolin. 1982. "Salpingectomy for Ectopic Pregnancy in the Sole Patient Oviduct: Reproductive Outcome." Fertility and Sterility 37:619.

Elias, S., M. LeBeau, J. L. Simpson, and A. O. Martin. 1981. "Chromosome Analysis of Ectopic Human Conceptuses." American Journal of Obstetrics and Gynecology 141:698.

Franklin, E. W., A. M. Zeiderman, and P. Laemmle. 1973. "Tubal Ectopic Pregnancy: Etiology and Obstetric and Gynecologic Sequelae." American Journal of Obstetrics and Gynecology 117: 220.

Honore, C. H. 1979. "A Significant Association between Spontaneous Abortion and Tubal Ectopic Pregnancy." Fertility and Sterility 32:401.

Kadar, N., G. Devare, and R. Romero. 1981. "Discriminatory HCG Zone: Its Use in the Sonographic Evaluation for Ectopic Pregnancy." Obstetrics and Gynecology 58:156.

Kitchen, J. D., R. M. Wein, W. C. Nunley, S. Thiagarajah, and W. N. Thornton. 1979. "Ectopic Pregnancy: Current Clinical Trends." American Journal of Obstetrics and Gynecology 134: 870.

Langer, R., I. Bukovsky, A. Herman, D. Sherman, G. Sadovsky, and E. Caspi. 1982. "Conservative Surgery for Tubal Pregnancy." Fertility and Sterility 38: 427.

Lundstrom, V., K. Bremme, P. Eneroth, I. Nygard, and M. Sundvall. 1979. "Serum Beta-Human Chorionic Gonadotrophin Levels in the Early Diagnosis of Ectopic Pregnancy." ACTA Obstetrics and Gynecology of Scandinavia 58:231.

Malhotra, N., and R. R. Chaudhwy. 1982. "Current Status of Intrauterine Devices. II. Intrauterine Devices and Pelvic Inflammatory Disease and Ectopic Pregnancy." Obstetrics and Gynecology Survey 37: 1.

Rosenfeld, D. L., and R. A. Bronson. 1980. "Reproductive Problems in the DES-Exposed Female." Obstetrics and Gynecology 55:453.

Rosenfeld, D. L., and E. Mitchell. 1979. "Treating the Emotional Aspects of Infertility: Counseling Services in an Infertility Clinic." American Journal of Obstetrics and Gynecology 135: 177.

Schenker, J. G., R. Eyal, and W. Z. Polishuk. 1972. "Fertility after Tubal Pregnancy." Surgery, Gynecology, and Obstetrics 135:74.

Schwartz, R. O., and D. L. DiPietro. 1980. "Beta-HCG as a Diagnostic Aid for Suspected Ectopic Pregnancy." Obstetrics and Gynecology 56:197.

Sherman, D., R. Langer, G. Sadovsky, I. Pukvosky, and E. Capsi. 1982. "Improved Fertility following Ectopic Pregnancy." Fertility and Sterility 37:497.

Thibault, C. 1972. "Some Pathological Aspects of Ovum Maturation and Gamete Transport in Mammals and Man." ACTA Endocrinology (supplement) 166:59.

Westrum, L. 1980. "Incidence, Prevalence and Trends of Acute Pelvic Inflammatory Disease and Its Consequences in Industrialized Countries." American Journal of Obstetrics and Gynecology 138:88.

14

The Abortion Experience in Private Practice

*David H. Sherman,
Nathan Mandelman,
Thomas D. Kerenyi,
and Jonathan Scher*

The elective termination of pregnancy has become a major service provided by gynecologists in the United States since the 1973
Supreme Court decision allowing abortion. The decision to abort an
unwanted or an unanticipated pregnancy (or a pregnancy that cannot
be followed to completion, for a host of possible reasons) has been
faced and made by an increasing number of women and important
others over the intervening years. Available statistics are based only
upon legal abortions that are reported to the appropriate agencies.
A significant number of abortions that are performed legally and safely
in private offices go unnoted. At a minimum, 33 percent of pregnant
women now terminate their pregnancies, resulting in approximately
2 million abortions per year in the United States. The technical procedures devised and perfected to carry them out, up to the generally
legal 24th week of gestation, have proved to be physically safe. Significantly less than 1 woman per 100,000 dies from elective abortion
(U.S., Department of Health and Human Services 1980).

Few medical procedures and issues have become embroiled in
so many arenas. The issue of abortion is debated from religious,
moral, political, legal, philosophical, and social perspectives. The
connotative context in which abortion has been maintained has powerful effects on the experience of all involved—the woman who makes
the choice, her partner and family, the physician, and the other ser-
vice-providing health professionals. Indeed, society as a whole
seems to be grappling with the issue (Adler 1980). It is possible that
women might again be denied this freedom of choice.

The authors acknowledge with much appreciation the contributions of Evelyn Horn, M.D., and Natalie Roche, M.D., medical students who conducted the interviews.

Approximately one-third of the abortions performed each year in the United States are carried out by private practitioners at the request of their patients. Although literature from before and after the legalization of abortion is extensive, it does not contain a single study of the postabortion sequelae and attitudes of women specifically receiving gynecologic care in the private sector. Previously published abortion studies came solely from the most readily available population, women in the clinic setting. Many earlier reports reflect findings (1) from research conducted when abortion was illegal and/or under much stricter regulation and imbued with even more negative connotations than it is now; (2) from research conducted by psychiatrists, naturally on a much more selected group of women; and/or (3) from research reflecting the long-held and repetitively reported belief that significant psychiatric problems follow induced abortion. The individual populations studied, the medical, psychiatric, or societal circumstances surrounding the abortion, the bias of the researchers and the previous data that they may have relied upon may have been reflected in the results produced.

The works of Ekblad (1955) and Simon and Sentura (1967) confirmed that references to postabortive psychiatric illness were unfounded. We may now firmly conclude that gynecologists are not socially and legally granting a right, nor are we medically partaking in an action that will cause women to decompensate or to become seriously ill in a psychiatric or even medical sense.

Some of the more recent literature has tended to the other extreme, that is, to stress the benignness of elective abortion and almost to minimize its effects upon the woman. A change in bias may have taken place, perhaps to add support to the liberalization of the abortion law. There seems to be satisfaction in reporting that severe psychological reactions simply do not occur. Many studies seem to ignore the significance of the reactions that are reported. Others report "negative" responses but stress how rapidly they are resolved and that they are not of sufficient frequency or intensity to create problems for most women who have undergone abortions.

The authors of this chapter regard the provision of abortion services and the maintenance of its availability to those who wish or need to avail themselves of it as an essential part of the practice of obstetrics and gynecology. Indeed, a possible change in the law might raise significant legal and ethical problems for them, since the continuation of what they consider to be complete, vital, and necessary services might be restricted.

Both before and after the time of legalization, the authors have witnessed, treated, counseled, experienced, and indeed sometimes shared the emotions surrounding the event with the patients. We have long been aware of the fact that an elective abortion, even remote to the moment, seems to cast a cloud of reluctance to recall it upon the patient who relates it as part of her initial history. We wished to explore in greater depth this usually elective endeavor, its meaning to the woman, and her response to it.

A questionnaire was developed, which was to be administered in the form of an interview by two female medical students. It was designed to furnish demographic data, information about contraceptive use, circumstances surrounding the need to abort, pre- and post-abortion attitudes and feelings, and general attitudes about abortion.

The purpose of the study was to evaluate some of the short- and long-term effects of the abortion experience as subjectively related by women who had had an abortion. The investigation was descriptive and was conducted in our private offices. The setting was unusual, and the data we collected were important because previous research on abortion attitudes and experiences had been conducted exclusively at clinics, hospitals, and public agencies.

According to a pilot study conducted previously by members of the community medicine department of the Mount Sinai School of Medicine (Safrin 1981), the population was rather uniform regarding education, socioeconomic background, availability of gynecologic care, knowledge relative to contraception, and satisfaction with the gynecologist and gynecologic care.

The questionnaire and interviews in our study were based on the following hypotheses:

1. That abortion is a major decision and crisis in the lives of most women;
2. That women's attitudes on the issue of abortion may change after having personally experienced one;
3. That having an abortion often results in changes in various aspects of women's lives including male-female relationships and the method of contraception used;
4. That despite the adverse effects encountered with having the abortion, most women would choose to make the same decision again;
5. That the legalization of abortion has not made it a light undertaking that is used thoughtlessly for birth control;
6. That women who have aborted would still consider this procedure to be a viable alternative to an additional unwanted pregnancy.

In addition, we were interested in gaining whatever subjective responses were offered as an evaluation of the woman's emotional reactions to the abortion.

Each morning of the interviews, the charts of all patients with appointments that day were reviewed to identify those who had had abortions. All patients showing up for repeat visits with such a history were asked to voluntarily participate in the study. There was no selective screening and all of the women who were approached agreed to participate. Interviews were conducted in private by both of the women medical students, and each interview lasted from 20 to 30 minutes. One hundred women with a combined history of 124 induced abortions were studied with this semistructured interview schedule.

The limitations of the study are obvious. The population was rather small and, certainly, select. The premise upon which the questionnaire was based may reflect bias, and the study was much more descriptive than it was statistical. Nevertheless, we believe that it illuminates several very important issues. Some very distinct differences from previously reported results were found, certain groups of women were identified who are at greater risk for emotional stress, and pertinent recommendations were made to private practitioners so that (1) they may better understand the reaction to abortion and (2) they may identify patients who might benefit from added support or assistance.

The population was quite different from any previously reported upon in the literature: 79 percent of the abortions took place after the age of 21, 75 percent of the women were either married or had a long-term ongoing relationship at the time of the termination, and all of the women questioned admitted to knowledge about contraception and had easy access to medical care. The population was 80 percent white and essentially equally divided in terms of religion, 66 percent had at least an undergraduate college degree, 71 percent were employed full-time, and 57 percent had an income over $20,000 per year. This was certainly not the young, poor, nonwhite, and unmarried group most often reported upon in the literature. The vast majority of these women (81 percent) had had one abortion; 14 percent, two; and 5 percent, three. In terms of gestation, the group was essentially equally divided into thirds: one-third had had a pregnancy before an abortion, one-third had had a child since aborting, and one-third had had an abortion or abortions representing the sole content of their obstetrical history. Of the total group of participants, 71 percent stated that they planned to have children in the future.

Choosing to terminate the pregnancy represented a major decision in the lives of most of these women: 62 percent directly responded in the affirmative when asked that question, 46 percent agreed that the abortion represented a major crisis in their lives, and another 5 percent felt that it was still too early to tell. A significant number of women who told us that they did not perceive the abortion as being a major decision revealed during the interview that they so responded only because they had no alternatives. For most of these women, however, the events surrounding the abortion were major. Relationships were suddenly and unexpectedly shaken; family and financial pressures arose; and for some, personal or family illness dictated the termination. Although only 5 percent of the pregnancies were planned, many of the women recalled significant ambivalence about termination. Many wished that their situation had been different and that they could have had the child. Many felt angry about having to abort. Women with Catholic backgrounds and those who had had a previous abortion more frequently expressed thoughts implying infanticide to abortion. The conceptus was often referred to as a baby, and some envisioned it as a real child. Calculated birth dates were sometimes remembered. Of those interviewed, 48 percent believed that the relationship they had with their male partners was in some way significantly altered by the abortion (this was approximately equally split, positive and negative). Thirty-three percent felt that their sexual performance (enjoyment or ease of forming a relationship) had been negatively affected to some degree. Two women considered themselves to be sexually incapacitated. Fifty-two percent were reluctant to have people find out that they had had an abortion, and 5 percent would only tell a gynecologist about it (that is, no other physician). The events, the emotional impact, and the circumstances surrounding the abortion were vividly recalled by the majority. Only 7 percent have sought psychological counseling for any reason since the abortion, and none had been psychiatrically hospitalized.

Statistically, we would conclude that elective abortion does not represent an act lightly undertaken by the majority of women, that it represents a major decision in the lives of most, and that the events surrounding the need to terminate a pregnancy were frequently recalled as a time of crisis. Varying degrees of ambivalence, confusion, anger, regret, and loss were felt by most. Emotionally charged memories exist in almost all, and the event was associated with objective changes in the lives of many.

In contrast to previous studies (Adler 1975; Brody, Meikle, and Gerritse 1971), the feeling of relief—although common—was by no means the major initial response to the gestation's termination. Often cited in previous studies, recalled feelings of joy, happiness, or freedom were relatively uncommon among this group of women. During the first month after the abortion, as many women recalled feeling sadness, a sense of significant loss, and/or an emptiness as recalled sensing relief and happiness. Almost twice as many experienced guilt, anger, anxiety, and/or confusion. A significant number had bad dreams, a fear of retribution, and the anxiety of being sterile in the future. No women ever expressed the feeling of joy. Recalled emotions relative to the abortion were reduced by some 75 percent during the second to sixth month afterward. More than two-thirds of those women who initially experienced relief and happiness no longer recalled those feelings. At this point, as many women still recalled feeling sad as those who felt relief. Although residual emotions were substantially diminished with time, the most often recalled remaining feelings were still guilt, anger, anxiety, confusion, and/or a fear of sterility. During the second six months, conscious feelings continued to diminish. Only 3 percent still felt relief, but 5 percent still felt anger, sadness, confusion, anxiety, and/or the need to forget. Freedom, a feeling not described by any of the women in the preceding months, was now reported by 5 percent. Obviously, an emergence was taking place.

Clearly, most of these women experienced a constellation of feelings commonly associated with death and a significant loss. A distinct period of bereavement took place. These associated emotions, although called negative ones in some previous reports, were indeed the norm in this study. Perhaps they should be viewed as necessary and positive ones in the process of successfully resolving the ambivalence that most women feel about terminating a pregnancy. The period of mourning was short for most. The feelings, although soon suppressed, were responsible for most women remembering the abortion as a very sad event in their lives.

For the vast majority of these women, the stated need to abort fell into a well-known list of generally socially acceptable reasons. The commonest, of course, was being unwed; financial difficulties were next; and then age, educational or career planning, being married too recently, a very young child at home, too many other children, and an unstable marital or social relationship followed. A few women declared that they would never want to have a child. Two women aborted because of diagnosed genetic or developmental abnormalities of the fetus. Three blamed the decision purely upon family pressures. Three aborted because of a serious illness recently diagnosed in themselves or their spouse. One chose to abort because she had taken large doses of tranquilizers before she realized that she was pregnant.

Although most women experienced at least some degree of ambivalence (and some a great deal about the choice that they had made), very few of them seriously questioned the validity of the reasons for which they chose to terminate. In general, the action was viewed merely as a delaying of ultimately having desired children. None of the women we interviewed saw at the time or admitted to later seeing a viable alternative to the choice they made. It is interesting that in spite of this recalled and declared resoluteness, 95 percent stated that abortion counseling should be available to women having an abortion, and 9.5 percent stated that they would not have an abortion if faced with an unwanted pregnancy in the future. A less-than-conscious or poorly suppressed question about their actions must continue to exist.

It became obvious that the mature and psychologically healthy woman—who could clearly and firmly rationalize her reasons to abort upon a socially acceptable basis, while feeling that she was merely delaying ultimately having a family—fared the best. It then became clear that when this set of circumstances was different, the experienced sense of loss and mourning seemed to increase substantially.

Although this study included only a few women who had abortions during their early teens, they generally seemed to recall stronger, negative, internally based emotions. These residua of substantial loss may have been generated because teenagers have less ability to foresee their potential autonomy and realistic future (Hatcher 1976). Most recalled that the abortion was essentially forced upon them.

The single woman, 35 years or older, unmarried or with an unstable social situation, experienced a greater sense of loss, disappointment, and a myriad of emotions usually associated with death and mourning. This group requires significant and understanding counseling and, we believe, is at risk for ongoing symptoms of remorse and depression. To these women the termination often seems, consciously or unconsciously, to be viewed as most likely an end to long-held desires and dreams, not merely as a holding action. Seemingly shattered fantasies of marriage and family add a serious burden to an event already documented to be sad. More than a fetus may have died and is being mourned. It is our clinical observation, other than from this study, that unless some positive social change occurs within a short period of time in the lives of these women, they remain somewhat chronically saddened by the need to have aborted.

Women previously indoctrinated with a traditional Catholic background are seemingly less able to successfully rationalize their actions. They are, therefore, at greater risk for suffering residua of their choice. This group must also be watched and counseled. Their potential feelings must be explored by the physician who offers the service of terminating the unwanted pregnancy. Of the small percentage of women in this study who subsequently sought psychiatric help and from our own general clinical experience, we have found that the longest-lasting depression and need for professional help occurs in the group of Catholic women who have an abortion in their mid-twenties without a permanent or meaningful relationship.

The group of recidivist aborters generally experienced some added difficulty in making the subsequent decision or decisions. Obviously, poorly resolved emotions surfaced and compounded their present predicament. It is within this group of women that we found a new emotion, perhaps a necessary rationalization for doing it again: there was often a verbalized relief in the reaffirmation of their fertility. Several even suggested that they may have tried to get pregnant in order to test their reproductive capabilities. Some of the sadness was replaced, at least consciously and temporarily, by this thought and emotion. Perhaps physicians should even point out this

potentially positive feature to women suffering obviously painful ambivalence in making a decision about which they may have no real alternative.

The sequelae of selective abortion, the termination of a planned
and wanted pregnancy because of diagnosed chromosomal or developmental abnormalities, has been addressed in the medical literature
(Kalinich 1982, Powledge and Fletcher 1979). The two patients in our
study, who were interviewed in depth, experienced significant initial
depression and lingering manifestations of anger, sadness, fear, and
anxiety. Events surrounding the termination have led to the disruption of one of the marriages, and the other woman is at present sec-
ondarily sterile, probably of psychological etiology. This type of
abortion is clearly complicated by the fact that it usually must be done
in mid-trimester and long following the rejoicing and perception of
actual fetal movement. The loss is obvious. Less obvious, however,
may be (1) the shame in having produced a defective child, (2) the
guilt relative to feeling that perhaps they chose the easy way out, and
(3) obviously, the real fears and anxieties relative to the normalcy
of future conceptions. The successful resolution of what is generally
a short mourning process is complicated and disrupted by these issues. Genetic and/or obstetrical departments, who have developed
the capabilities of making these diagnoses, must now develop the ability to counsel these women in a multidisciplinary fashion. In general,
this has not been addressed. We would also suggest that a support
network of women who have gone through the experience be established,
which can be called upon to assist couples through the abortion/mourn-
ing period.

Women who must abort because of a serious illness in self or
spouse may also require knowledgeable counseling. They may best
be viewed as a subgroup within the population requiring selective abortion. Their loss and bereavement are also obviously complicated by
the fact that future children might be affected and/or not possible.
This group is frightened, frequently expresses anger, and clearly,
feel potentially cheated.

Women who must opt for abortion because they inadvertently
took drugs or teratogenic medications before realizing that they were
pregnant often experience loss complicated by significant guilt. The
physician must be careful not to parentally lecture or chide; advice
and recommendations for the future are much more appropriate and
therapeutic.

Despite the current trend toward minimizing the negative feelings of women who undergo voluntary abortion, there are many women
who are vulnerable to suffering from anxiety, guilt, and depression as
sequelae of thus terminating a pregnancy. We have elucidated those
groups of women who are at greater risk for an exaggerated emotional

response and for the possibility of long-lasting difficulties. There is definitely a small number of women who will require psychological treatment or counseling afterward.

Preabortion counseling by the physician and/or a trained member of the office staff is necessary. Under ordinary circumstances, it may be simple and rather brief and yet be effective. Although rarely chosen, it still must include an exploration of possible alternatives. An attempt must be made to include the spouse or the significant other in the decision-making process. Someone else should at least be included to share the physical pain and emotional discomfort later, since women who abort alone do not seem to fare as well emotionally as women who share the experience. The physician and staff must project a caring and understanding affect. By actions, words, or atmosphere, the importance of the decision that the patient is forced to make must not be taken lightly. Although morbidness is clearly uncalled for, a dignity appropriate to the action is required. Certainly, a judgmental attitude must be avoided at all costs. The reasons, albeit perhaps rationalized, for terminating the pregnancy should probably be reinforced if ambivalence seems to be a significant problem. If the patient falls within a group of women at greater risk, a discussion of possible reactions should be initiated and she should be told that someone will be available to help should she need it. The time between making the decision and undergoing the procedure should be as short as possible in order to reduce anxiety and the omnipresent ambivalence. Delay seems to serve no purpose relative to a change of mind. Naturally, future contraception must be promoted. The procedure itself should be described in as much detail as the patient seems to want to be told or to know about. Some women do not wish to be told, and others seem to require more details in order to allay physical fears. A brief anatomy lesson may, at times, be in order. Even among educated women, misunderstandings are not unusual. The continuation of fertility following an uneventful abortion should be stressed, since many women fear the possibility of infertility or even retribution.

In conclusion, although the results of our study may not be surprising, this may be an important time to reiterate them, because we face a potential change in the status of legal abortion. Sadness and bereavement did not change the attitude of women who experienced abortion: 90.5 percent said that they would do it again if it became necessary. All said that they hoped it would not be necessary. Freedom of choice must not be denied on the basis of the fact that moral women react appropriately after they have made a decision to end a potential life. The fact that most of the women we studied experienced loss and grief rather than joy and freedom is, perhaps, an affirmation of the goodness of mankind rather than the wrongness of abortion.

All choices are not simple; consequences of free will exist, but we must not limit choices because of the normal emotions they evoke.

REFERENCES

Adler, N. 1980. "Psychosocial Issues of Therapeutic Abortion."
In Psychosomatic Obstetrics and Gynecology, edited by D. D.
Youngs and A. Elmhardt, pp. 159-77. New York: Appleton-
Century-Crofts.

Adler, N. E. 1975. "Emotional Responses of Women following
Therapeutic Abortion." American Journal of Orthopsychology
45:446-54.

Brody, H., S. Meikle, and R. Gerritse. 1971. "Therapeutic Abortion: A Prospective Study." American Journal of Obstetrics
and Gynecology 109: 347-52.

Ekblad, N. 1955. "Induced Abortion on Psychiatric Grounds."
ACTA Psychiatric Scandinavia (supplement).

Hatcher, S. 1976. "Understanding Adolescent Pregnancy and Abortion." Primary Care 3:407-25.

Kalinich, L. J. 1982. "The Management of the Female Patient."
In Psychiatric Management for Medical Practitioners, edited
by D. S. Kornfeld and J. B. Finkel, pp. 61-85. New York:
Grune & Stratton.

Powledge, M. S., and J. Fletcher. 1979. "Guidelines for the Ethical,
Social, and Legal Issues in Prenatal Diagnosis." New England
Journal of Medicine 300: 168-72.

Safrin, D. 1981. "Dysmenorrhea and the Premenstrual Syndrome:
A Descriptive Study." Unpublished manuscript.

Simon, N., and D. Sentura. 1967. "Psychiatric Illness following
Therapeutic Abortion." American Journal of Psychology 124:1.

U.S., Department of Health and Human Services. 1980. Abortion
Surveillance. Centers for Disease Control, annual summary.

15

Death of a Newborn: Immediate and Long-term Effects on the Family

Gladys B. Lipkin

A neonatal death represents a catastrophic situation for families. The body may be small, but the loss is never trivial to those who are involved. The U.S. Department of Health and Human Services has estimated that 45,000 infants died in 1980, which translates into an infant mortality rate of 12.5 deaths per 1,000 live births. The fact that this is the lowest annual rate ever noted in this country is of small comfort to the parents of those children who died, whether as stillborns or after a live birth.

The death of a newborn is rarely anticipated. It almost always comes as a shock, finding parents and relatives unprepared to cope. Their individual mechanisms for handling grief may vary considerably, from crying and sharing with others to quiet and self-isolation. Some mourners even put up a cheerful front when they are with others, to "protect" them from realizing the depths of the inner pain being felt. This public denial of feeling often prolongs the time needed to work through the grief involved in the loss.

Silence really has no place in the care of a mother who leaves the hospital without a baby, particularly if the baby has little chance for survival. The same holds true if the infant dies after discharge from the hospital. Instead, feelings about this and future pregnancies should be recognized, verbalized, and acknowledged. Parents need support and understanding, and they often require professional help in order to communicate their hurts and fears to each other—and eventually to resolve them. They may also need help in preparing to deal with the inevitable questions and comments from outsiders once their loss is made known. Above all, they may need permission to cry and be angry.

Whenever possible, staff members should be available to relatives of newborns who are unlikely to survive. At first, the parents or others may only be able to use nonverbal communication, perhaps clinging to, stroking, or holding each other. They may cry, sob, or even scream as the enormity of the situation is recognized. These expressions of feelings should be encouraged, since they certainly are appropriate. This is not the time for intellectualizing or sedating, but rather, for an honest expression of gut-level emotions. Staff members should find a place where emotional outbursts do not have to be hushed, where no one has to feel inhibited about expressing or sharing feelings. Parents should also be offered the chance to spend time with the baby and receive answers to their questions. Whenever possible, the mother should be asked whether she wants to be placed on a postpartum floor, where babies will visit with their parents, or whether she prefers to be on another floor. It is usually advantageous, although painful, for her to remain on the postpartum unit, where nurses are generally more supportive and comfortable with grieving mothers.

Verbal communication between family members is important. It may be difficult to establish, since each one may be silent in an effort to protect the others from a deepening of emotional wounds. In fact, the silence causes an even bigger wound, with the unexpressed feelings of hurt often brought out through tangential issues. This may result in angry arguments about unconnected events, the use of mind-altering drugs to ease the pain, or other tactics to avoid or deny the issue at hand. There may be difficulty in reaching out to one another, giving or receiving comfort, or sharing concerns about present and future events. The earlier communication starts, the easier it is to prevent estrangement.

Mothers may find their sleep patterns interrupted by nightmares about the baby and may be reluctant to share these or the sense of unreality that may be present during the days following the delivery. During the last trimester of pregnancy, the mother may have had dreams about defective or dead babies. Unless she is told that those were just normal expressions of prebirth anxiety, she may believe that they were warnings of what was to come. If so, similar dreams during future pregnancies will cause her to expect another infant death. In addition, she should be told that many mothers have feelings of unreality following normal deliveries, and that the death was not a punishment for her lack of emotional attachment to the newborn. Again, if this is not done, she may have emotional difficulty following future deliveries, since there is likely to be an even longer delay between the birth and attachment to the newborn. This occurs in response to the fear that this baby, too, may not survive.

Mothers also have to deal with the changes in body image. The physical expansion during pregnancy may have been disturbing, but it was probably accepted because it meant there would be a baby. Those bodily changes now represent a negative experience, with some permanent changes acting as a constant reminder. The red stretch marks on the abdomen are one such reminder of what might have been, and they will remain so even when they fade. The same feelings are evoked by the episiotomy, the bloody lochia, and the swollen breasts, which may even produce milk for the baby who will never suckle.

The mother may have a scar from a cesarean section as permanent proof of the space that she once provided to nurture another being, one whom she can never hold or touch again. But her love for the baby may still be very real, and she will need help in changing that into a positive feeling without the constant association of painful loss.

The immediate reactions of parents after the infant's death usually include numbness, shock, overwhelming grief, guilt, anger, and a sense of failure for producing an imperfect child. Anger may be expressed at God for having taken the child or even at the baby for causing them so much pain. In multiple births, where one or more of the infants have died, there may be anger at the survivor(s) for not having shared sufficient oxygen, nutrients, or whatever with the one(s) who died. And there may be anger at the world because this experience is costing so much money. There may not be any logical reasons for these feelings. However, it is unwise to focus on logic at this time. It is more important to provide support and to encourage verbalization.

Whether or not they have received a specific reason for what has happened, parents often regard the death as punishment for their own or partner's past errors. Those who have terminated previous pregnancies, had extramarital affairs, or were involved in any past indiscretions, may look upon the death as a penalty for those offenses. They may not accept any reassurance that their misdeed did not play a role. It is pointless to argue, because feelings, rather than logic, have taken over. Genetic counseling may be helpful in determining whether subsequent pregnancies are likely to have similar outcomes, but it will have no bearing on the parents' expression of guilt. One offshoot of this guilt may be an inability for the parents to enjoy life in the future, thereby punishing themselves. This may include a refusal to give or receive love in any form, leading to sexual problems.

Anger about the death may be displaced onto anyone involved in the care of either the mother or infant. It is not unusual for family members to criticize the level of professional care received, performance of the care givers, hospital accommodations, food, or anything else that comes to mind. Professionals may become defensive as they become the butt of the anger. It is difficult not to be uncomfortable in such a situation, particularly if the highest possible level of care has been provided and is deemed unacceptable by the family. Innocent statements by professionals may be distorted and may feed into the family's belief that the care was inadequate. Physicians, nurses, social workers, psychologists, and the institution itself may all share the ill will of the family. There is less likelihood of this occurring when the staff establishes rapport with the patient and family.

Even though the baby may be born dead, the sense of loss is overwhelming. During the pregnancy, parents work to integrate the new person into their lives, and now the space they have provided remains unfilled. It is as though they have snatched and lost a valuable prize at the same time. The loss is profound. Future children will not (and should not be expected to) fill the void. This baby has a unique place, one that is etched into the minds of parents forever. The loss will be felt in the future on the actual date of birth, and even perhaps on the expected date of delivery, as well as during family celebrations and holidays.

Since society as a whole has difficulty in dealing with the death of a newborn, it may be treated as a nonevent. Often the baby is not mentioned, and family and friends may even withdraw from the parents, fearing that whatever they say may intensify the pain of the loss. That fear is more likely to be an expression of their own uneasiness in a situation for which most people are unprepared. As outsiders resist being drawn into the drama, parents find few with whom to share their feelings. The lack of adequate outlets results in intensification of feelings of loss, anger, and isolation. Unless families, particularly mothers, are allowed to grieve, they may become candidates for multiple physical and emotional health problems.

Dreams often disturb the sleep patterns of bereaved parents. Many times the dreams involve searching closets, rooms, tunnels, or other areas for some unknown object. Interpretation, of course, is that they are searching for the missing child. This dream is often more intense among those parents who did not make burial plans for the infant or those who did not have the opportunity to see, touch, or hold the infant.

Most parents welcome the chance to examine the newborn, even in death, often trying to memorize the baby's features for future recall. Some ask for a photograph or for a list of vital statistics (weight, length, coloring, time of birth) as though trying to ensure that an indelible picture of the infant will remain in their minds. Some hospitals have already instituted a permanent file with this information, so that it will be available to parents at any time. This gives the baby substance and an identity. It also is helpful for the parents to select a name for the baby, to preserve his identity.

Some parents are unable to find an outlet for their grief, and so they internalize their feelings. Severe depression may then occur. Other illnesses may crop up fairly soon or even years later in response to the loss. Sometimes another event, even a death, triggers feelings that could not be expressed previously, leading to a physical or emotional upheaval. A subsequent normal birth may also result in a resurrection of old memories if the loss has not been resolved. Some parents, particularly mothers, express anger at the new, healthy child for interfering with memories of the lost infant. The fear of losing those memories becomes intensified unless, even at this late date, the previous losses are reexamined and discussed with an effort at resolution. The reaction may be so far removed in time from the original loss of the newborn that the relationship to the emotional stress may not be apparent immediately. For this reason, it is important to include a psychosocial history as part of the initial interview of every patient, regardless of the presenting symptoms.

Patients may seek treatment for depression or anxiety even decades after the death of the newborn, unaware of the psychic toll to which they have been subjected through the years. Others may document episodes of major or minor physical symptoms, including chest pains, heart palpitations, dizziness, eating disturbances, abnormal sleep patterns, inability to enjoy lovemaking, and lack of energy. As the history unfolds, the death may be mentioned casually, but purposeful questions encourage the surfacing of the hidden feelings. Most patients are then eager to share their memories. The inclusion of very minute details is an indication of how traumatic the event was and how much alive the issue remains.

The period of time between the birth and death of the infant may demand many decisions by the parents. Although theoretically they have the right to withhold permission for treatment, they may find their wishes ignored. At times, legal proceedings by the hospital or outsiders result in court orders to provide treatment against the express desires of the parents. This may lead to extreme bitterness, as the child is subjected to procedures that may be not only painful but fruitless and expensive. Support from staff members can help the parents discover and use any available options for care. They may find comfort in helping to decide when or where some treatments or procedures should take place. Incorporating their suggestions about care will help them achieve some sense of control of the child's destiny, thus regaining at least part of their parental rights.

When medical intervention is finally stopped, the family will need ongoing support as the focus changes from hope of life to that of impending death. Adults are not the only ones who are affected by an infant's demise. Children in the family may be going through similar turmoil, although their feelings may not be acknowledged by the grownups. In fact, youngsters have to deal with more than the death, for their parents often withdraw in response to their own unspeakable pain. This means that mothers and fathers are not available to provide comfort at a time when they are desperately needed.

How much should children be told about the death of a newborn?
Even without being told, they probably know a great deal. They can
sense the tension, see the tears of their parents and others. They
may feel isolated and displaced if they are not included in the sharing
of the event.

In the egocentricity and sense of omnipotence of childhood, siblings may be overwhelmed by feelings of guilt that their thoughts,
wishes, or actions caused the death, particularly if they did not want
a new baby in the family. This sense of somehow being responsible
may result in lifelong emotional problems unless they are helped to
verbalize their version of what happened, so that misconceptions can
be rectified before becoming ingrained. Children also need to share
in the sorrow, lest adult agony be interpreted as rejection.

Participation of siblings in a funeral, burial, or other services
provides a time and place for grieving. They may benefit by helping
to choose the clothing, blankets, or other items that will be with the
baby at burial. Family members can console one another and give
the children a sense of security. The message can be imparted that
the family unit was together before the death, is together in their bereavement, and will survive this trial and be together in the future.
How much more positive this is than relegating siblings to a nonpar-
ticipatory role. They should be encouraged to cry openly, without
fear of upsetting parents or others with their tears.

This may be a sibling's first experience with death. The child
may not be able to grasp the concept that the newborn will not be in
the home. He may overhear parents discussing the "loss" of the newborn and wonder whether there is a chance that he, too, may be "lost"
—or whether his parents may be "lost." Considering that very real
fear, is it any wonder that surviving children cling to their parents?

If surviving children are told that God needed an angel and took
the newborn to heaven, they may equate goodness with illness and
death. Perhaps virtue is dangerous. God is not likely to want trouble-
makers; therefore it may be safer to misbehave. Small wonder, then,
if "good" children change drastically in their behavior. In essence,
children are better off when given honest information to the extent of
their ability to understand.

Parents are usually very touchy during the immediate period
following the death. They often perceive statements by relatives,
friends, or even professionals as being unthinking, uncaring, unhelp-
ful, callous, or downright stupid. This is particularly true of comments implying that the mother did not take sufficient care of herself
during the pregnancy or that her health care providers were not competent.

It is less than therapeutic to suggest that parents forget the experience and get on with their lives. They may be young and they may
bear many more children, but they will not forget this child, nor are

they likely to cease mourning the loss. Although some literature states that resolution of the loss usually occurs in 18 to 24 months, most parents never fully put their grief to rest. Tears may come in response to losses suffered by others, on anniversary dates, or during happy celebrations that might have involved their child.

If the death involves a child of a multiple birth, outsiders usually focus on the live survivors. In contrast, the parents usually focus on the pain of loss. This is often incomprehensible to others. For comparison, if an individual loses a finger, or an arm, or a leg, or an eye, should he be asked to be grateful that he has nine other fingers, or another arm, leg, or eye? Does society ask her to ignore her loss? Can she ignore the lost part just because she has similar others? Why then should a parent be asked to ignore an infant that has been integrated into the family picture and then lost? The multiple birth was accepted as a package deal, and part of the package has been destroyed. Clothes and equipment may have been purchased, perhaps a move to a larger home has taken place. And now the need is gone.

Sharing the loss of the newborn can bring parents closer together emotionally if they are able to express their feelings to one another. Unfortunately, many are unable to do so, fearing that any show of sadness will increase the grief of the partner. This is far from the truth, for the mate who does not share is often seen as not caring. The pain then intensifies as each suffers alone. In situations where one parent has not wanted the pregnancy, the problem intensifies. The one who did not want the baby may be overwhelmed with guilt and grief, while the partner who wanted the baby may blame the other. If neither wanted the pregnancy, there may be mutual guilt and distress.

Another problem arises when one parent is further along in the mourning process and becomes impatient with the other. In some instances, the one who appears to have progressed faster (usually the father) may not have progressed at all, but still may be in a state of shock, unable to get in touch with any feelings. This discordance may lead to additional strain on the marital relationship, expressed through tangential arguments, a seeming lack of understanding or caring, and physical avoidance of each other.

At a time when the partners need closeness, tenderness, and mutual support, they may withdraw from each other sexually. This may be due to a need for self-punishment, to deny any comfort to themselves. They may, particularly the mothers, see themselves as unworthy of love because they have failed to protect the child through pregnancy, birth, and life. They may be fearful of becoming pregnant, resulting in another negative outcome, or they may view sexual pleasure as a desecration of the dead child's memory. Sexual involve-

ment is equated with life and living, and it may be unacceptable at
a time when all thoughts are of death. If a state of mutual or one-
sided rejection continues, the marriage may unravel and become dysfunctional. It is important for professionals to recognize this possibility and help the couple find a more acceptable way of demonstrating
their agony. This may well include professional counseling.

Future pregnancies are almost always accompanied by anxiety
concerning the outcome. No one can promise that the new pregnancy
will result in a healthy child. Parents need to express their concerns
and receive support from the health care providers. Some couples
may experience additional losses, perhaps never producing a baby
who can survive. Each loss must be acknowledged fully, and increased
feelings of incompetence, inadequacy, guilt, and anger must be vented.
The greater the number of losses, the more intense the reaction. No
one ever gets used to this kind of loss. Repetition only increases the
anguish.

It is important to realize that the newborn who dies is rarely
forgotten. His or her presence on earth, however brief, leaves an
indelible mark on the family. It is the task of care givers to help
families cope with the loss, so that the pain of their experience will
eventually resolve into a loving memory.

16

Unconscious Motivation in the Refusal to Have Children

Muriel G. Morris

Much is heard about women making a conscious choice either to have or not to have children. Scientific knowledge of ovulatory cycles and the availability of birth control methods and devices have contributed to the illusions that these decisions are truly in the conscious realm by providing the mechanics for their implementation. Popular ideologies that glorify the workplace, while devaluing the world of women and children, and the narcissistic investment in careers previously reserved for the idealized male tantalize women and foster doubt in the minds of many who are already ambivalent about having children, even to the point of suppressing ovulation in some. Psychoanalysis, on the other hand, can do much to expose and resolve the underlying conflicts in these women and to enable them to resume their psychic development, attain parenthood, and live out the later stages of their biological life cycle in a gratifying way.

This chapter places particular emphasis on women who are organically infertile on a psychological basis, although in my opinion, they are psychodynamically on a continuum with many women who are physically fertile but nevertheless refuse to have children. In fact, the patient described later in this chapter was both infertile and consciously intolerant of the idea of having a child.

The motives for parenthood are deeply rooted. Its innateness and desirability have been described by many authors. The three major contributors who stand out on this subject are Therese Benedek (1959), who described parenthood as a developmental phase, Helene Deutsch (1945), who emphasized the potential for a sense of immortality sought through parenthood; and Erik Erikson (1963), who conceptualized a stage of "generativity," without which there ensues "psychic stagnation." Although Erikson included sublimated forms of creativity in his meaning of the term <u>generativity</u>, others have emphasized the importance of the actual experience of becoming a parent in its enabling function of furthering a person's prospects of psychologically achieving this stage.

Although most people want and try to have children, a state of doubt is often experienced over this undertaking, harking back to early events with the mothering figures who influenced them during identification formation in childhood. The narcissism of the early days of life and its intrinsic conflicts are reflected clearly in the ancient legends of the Old Testament, wherein three of the first progenitors of the new nation were born after periods of uncertain fertility in their mothers. Sarah agonized over her inability to conceive Isaac; Rebekkah had to wait and pray a long time for Jacob; and Jacob's favorite wife, Rachel, had to employ magic to conceive Joseph, who was destined to become Jacob's favorite son. There are many other instances of delayed conceptions, including those of Samuel and Samson. The fathers in these cases already had many less-valued children born of devalued women, including Abraham's son Ishmael (born to Hagar) and Jacob's sons born to Leah.

Significantly, the mothers of the more highly valued sons had fantasies of greatness for these children, on whom the survival of a whole people was to depend. Although we now understand that these archaic legends belong to an earlier age and may, in fact, simply be the same story retold several times with the names changed, one might expect, nevertheless, that they tell us something meaningful about unconscious thoughts and their effects on somatic functioning: that the more infantile grandiosity that is invested in the fantasies of prospective parents, the more trouble they might be expected to have in succeeding to parenthood, psychically or somatically or even both. In all patients with psychosomatic illness, as in psychogenic or hypothalamic infertility, the psychodynamic conflicts belong to the earliest stages of life. During these stages the narcissistic attachments are not yet resolved; separation-individuation from the mother figure is not well established; fantasies of bodily functions are still rooted in primitive oral and anal conflicts consisting of incorporative, retentive, and expulsive tendencies; and aggression is still linked to sadistic fantasies and is readily liberated under stress and frustration.

In the fantasies of little girls who are smitten with their daddies and who look forward to marrying and having children with them one day, we see the seeds of omnipotent fantasies that, if not repudiated early enough in life, can lead later on to derangements in psychosexual functioning, anovulation, and other difficulties in carrying fetuses to term and having normal deliveries. More work must be done to elucidate the exact mechanisms translating psychic conflict into physical symptoms and organic illness. However, it is known that in early life the emotions are expressed in physiological terms via the autonomic nervous system. It is readily seen how patterns established during that period are reactivated under emotional conflict in later life and mediated to the body via the hypothalamus.

We are taught that there is a ripe ovum every 28 days from ages 15 to 44 in the average woman. This overly simplified statement indicates the ardent desire to believe in the perfection of the reproductive apparatus, despite the fact that everyone who studies it is aware of its many imperfections and unpredictable malfunctions. Women who try to conceive are horrified and dismayed when they find themselves going from month to month without success. They commonly feel distraught and threatened in their sense of having normal reproductive capacities, even when reassured that this lag is quite commonplace. The sense of loss is enormous in the woman who keeps trying without conceiving and who sees the cycles, years, and chances ticking by. Today's expression up against the clock aptly refers to this conflict. Such a case was noted by the Spanish writer Federico Garcia Lorca in his play about Yerma, a woman whose frustration at her inability to conceive a child leads regressively to such murderous rage that, at the end of the play, she turns against her husband with a knife. Whatever symbolic meanings the play was intended to convey, the author recognized the depth of a woman's pain when she feels this loss, not even realizing that she may unconsciously be suppressing her own ovulation.

CASE STUDY: MRS. A

Background

The case of Mrs. A illustrates the conscious and unconscious levels at which the psychogenically infertile woman operates. Mrs. A's psychoanalysis ultimately shifted the balance in her mental life, so that the rejection of her periods no longer served its purpose of unconscious compromise, thus allowing her to progress naturally and normally to pregnancy and motherhood.

Mrs. A entered analysis at the age of 32, upset about the recent death of her father, her mother's psychosis, and her failure at the defense of her doctoral dissertation. She was anxious and depressed about her career and every aspect of her personal life. She was undecided about staying in her marriage and was full of complaints about her husband's disorderliness, self-centeredness, and male superiority. She had all the stereotypic complaints of a woman with an inferiority complex; she hated her role yet clung to housekeeping chores and assumed a moral superiority for doing so. She insisted she could never have children because she already had her husband to take care of. She was afraid of failing as a mother or going crazy like her own paranoid mother. She cynically declared that she expected better feedback from pets than from children, and she already had pets. She characterized herself and her husband as sheepdogs. She had a large collection of stuffed animals, including life-sized ones, which she played with and tucked in at night the way little girls do with their dolls.

Noteworthy about the childhood family of Mrs. A was the fact that it bore the typical stigmata of families of anorexic patients. Mrs. A was of normal weight but had a fear of being fat, and she was pre-occupied and anxious about all aspects of food and overeating. Her mother also had been preoccupied with her figure, dieting, and being fat. The patient blamed her mother for overfeeding her in early child-hood, causing her to have a fat latency and dooming her to a lifetime of the fear of being fat. There were pathological levels of aggression in the family, including paranoia and ostracism. Ostracism was also symbolically achieved by tearing faces out of family photos. The family was perfectionist and hypermoral in many ways, yet loosely moral in many others. The mother overcontrolled the patient and in-duced a goody-goody compliance in her. The mother was intrusive and exhibitionist, and the father was voyeuristic in sexual matters. He read pornography and gave it to the patient to read. At the same time, there was a detachment in areas where active participation was needed to help the patient master skills adaptive for living. The pa-tient was overly stimulated sexually by the parents' behavior, yet she was rejected and neglected when she needed support in her own social development. In addition, the mother was an unhappy, embittered narcissistic woman, who hated her role as wife and mother, felt martyred by her family, and discouraged her guilt-ridden daughter from forming positive feminine identifications.

When I took Mrs. A's menstrual history, she had been cycling artificially on birth control pills for ten years. Despite being edu-cated with booklets and consciously looking forward to her menarche, she experienced only two cycles at age 14, followed by total cessation of her periods. In addition to menstrual problems, Mrs. A hated her breasts. She felt they were small and useless and would make suc-cess in life impossible. Unconsciously, success meant subjugation of the world at her feet and her father's enthrallment with her, simi-lar to his feelings toward her beautiful mother.

When she was 17, Mrs. A's mother took her for an inconclusive gynecological workup. This three-year lag in seeking help indicates the mother's self-absorption as well as more malignant attitudes to-ward the patient, including discouraging of maturation and showing disappointment that the patient was not a boy. Furthermore, she scuttled any positive attitudes from the workup by humiliating the patient in front of a friend, saying, "You can't go to the beach! You have to stay home and collect your urine!"

Over the years, the patient was subjected to confusing and exploitative treatment that undermined her strivings for femininity, independence, and initiative. Both parents interfered with her social life with men, the mother attacking her for kissing a boy on a date, the father lasciviously intruding with wisecracks—"Hey, did you sleep with him?" Mrs. A's inadequate wardrobe and ill-fitting brassiere when she went away to college were indicative of her unreadiness for young adulthood. It was in college that she realized she no longer wanted the baby she had desired all through her youth. She replaced that fantasy with the primary yearning for a diamond on her finger by graduation and a passive-dependent marital relationship.

In her early twenties Mrs. A sought medical advice, again inconclusively. The doctors gave her a cortisone shot, which brought on one period. Subsequently, she went on the birth control pill for the next ten years. At no time was psychoanalysis recommended nor was the patient told that her condition was psychophysiological. Only when her mother was certified as psychotic and her father died did she come for psychiatric help.

In the beginning of her psychoanalysis, Mrs. A was angry and demanding toward me for a redress of all her grievances. Her antipathy to having children showed a typical sour-grapes defense. Gradually over four years, as our relationship shifted to a more positive side, Mrs. A took more active responsibility for understanding and accepting her woman's body, as well as for acknowledging her yearning for ovulation and a baby. She engaged a male gynecologist, indicating her awareness that her mental and gonadal problems did not originate in the fantasied cruel, male-dominated external universe, but rather in her own mind. Step by step she gave up the pill, ovulated, and had her baby. An outline of the psychic conflicts and constellations that emerged and were worked on in Mrs. A's treatment shows how urgently she required a psychological approach, not just for her lost fertility but for her general well-being as well.

Psychodynamics

1. Mrs. A suppressed her ovulation because of extreme ambivalence about femininity.
2. She felt rage and envy toward men for their supposed advantages in life. She refused to share with her husband or to give him any credit.
3. She had almost delusional thinking about the wrongs of society, which were representations of her early relationship with her mother projected onto society.

4. She denied and refused any input that would correct her misconceptions because of lack of trust, anger, and fear of taking any risks. She suffered from an incapacity to tolerate ambiguities, stating that she preferred and felt safer with consistency, whether or not it represented an accurate picture of reality.

5. She lacked supportive input from a nurturing maternal figure about the specific pleasures and advantages of femininity and motherhood. Her mother had perceived these traits and functions as the cause of her own unhappiness and eventual psychosis.

6. Mrs. A had the fear of going crazy through identification with her narcissistic and, later, psychotic mother.

7. The patient continually experienced the painful effects of the threat of abandonment by an angry, withdrawn, and depressed maternal figure. She projected these representations onto other significant objects in her current life.

8. The patient suffered from an intense fear of death. As she put it, "When you have a child, you know you are going to die." She was afraid of intensifying her mother's pathological fear of death by growing up and having children herself.

9. She fantasized that she could magically stop the clock and keep her mother young forever by rejecting and denying the existence of her own adult woman's body. Her refusal to accept her breasts as adequate, her insistence that her hips were too large as part of a general concern about overweight, and her failure to ovulate were aspects of this rejection and denial.

10. Mrs. A demonstrated her moral superiority over her mother by refusing to have children, while her mother, on the other hand, who was incapable of taking good care of children, showed weakness by giving in to the desire to have them. This moral superiority gave Mrs. A a sense of compensation for her loss in not having children.

11. Mrs. A wished to stay on the good side of her needy mother, rather than to grow up and become independent of her.

12. Mrs. A treated other people as if she were on the verge of abandoning them, which was how her mother had treated her.

13. Mrs. A had magical beliefs in her own powers, which were never repudiated. She was angry at me because the analysis did not redress her grievances and I did not use the delegated omnipotence she bestowed upon me to correct the wrongs that had been done to her. Her attitude toward me was as follows: "You have to meet my infantile needs and stop depriving me, because I have given up everything for you," namely, her ovulation and a chance to have a baby in the somatic realm and her autonomy in the psychic realm.

14. Mrs. A's failure to ovulate and menstruate was further reinforced by her mother's disinterest in arranging for medical evaluation within an appropriate time limit.

15. Mrs. A played with dolls and pets as a continuation of her childhood play in which she fantasized being married to her father and having little doll and pet babies with him.

16. She lived in fear of retaliation from a hostile maternal figure as punishment for these oedipal wishes.

17. Mrs. A's fantasies about menstruation were related to oral and anal tendencies from early life. She thought that menstrual blood was a sign of internal damage and that it emerged without sphincter control as an excretory product while she was sitting on a toilet. Her fantasies about impregnation and birth were based on ideas of eating and excreting.

Only after the resolution of these unconscious conflicts could this patient move on to true generativity, psychic and somatic.

In many patients, efforts to force generativity by physical manipulations run the risk of being blocked by further psychic barriers or serious regressions. It has been noted that some patients whose organic problems are corrected still do not conceive, because of underlying psychological problems. Contrarily, it has also been determined that 14 percent of infertile adoptive couples progress to having their own biological children after the adoption.

CONCLUSION

In conclusion, the therapist's essential role must be mentioned. The therapist must recognize his or her own unconscious fantasies and constellations about the generative and later-life stages, being alert and ready to (1) recognize the unfolding psychological material referable to this theme and (2) interpret it systematically to these patients. The sense of timelessness that neurotic patients have because of the dominance of the primary process in their unconscious definitely works against these women. If they do not work to solve their problems within a reasonable time frame, they will be left with a sense of permanent loss. The loss will have to be mourned and this may lead to incomplete or failed treatment, with the therapist assigned the role (in the patients' minds) of the mother, who actually and unfortunately hindered their development in early life.

REFERENCES

Benedek, T. 1959. "Parenthood as a Developmental Phase." Journal of the American Psychoanalytic Association 7:389-417.

Deutsch, H. 1945. <u>The Psychology of Women</u>, vol. 2. New York: Grune & Stratton.

Erikson, E. H. 1963. "Eight Ages of Man." In <u>Childhood and Society</u>, rev. ed. New York: W. W. Norton.

Part III
Life-Threatening Illness and Body Image

17

Thanatological Aspects
of Maternal Mortality

William F. Finn

The death of a woman during pregnancy or at delivery is a shocking tragedy. Everyone—expectant mother, father, children, relatives, friends—is looking forward to a joyous event. Showers have been given and presents have been bought. The new baby's room has been painted and refurbished. Husband and wife leave for the hospital. Labor progresses. Then, unexpectedly, the woman in labor dies.

The father has waited outside the delivery room suite. The doctor walks out. The father's anticipation of joy bursts as the doctor says, "We could not save her." Still it has not dawned on the husband that the doctor is referring not to the baby but to his wife. Life and future go down the drain. He throws away the list of phone numbers to call. Where can he go? How can he tell the other children? How can he make the calls to his parents, in-laws, and relatives? How can he complete the mechanics of death—the funeral arrangements, the burial plot, the legal involvements? How can he care for the children? How can he support them when his heart is broken? How can he reorganize the family's life?

Maternal mortality, or death associated with pregnancy, is defined as any death occurring during pregnancy or within 90 days of the completion of pregnancy (American Medical Association 1964). Such deaths include abortions and ectopic pregnancies. Historically, deaths at term have been caused by hemorrhage, infection, and toxemia. Now, however, the most common causes of maternal death are ectopic pregnancies, general anesthesia, rupture of a cerebral vascular malformation, or cancer. Death can occur at any time during pregnancy and results in a double tragedy if the unborn child dies as well. If the death occurs close to term or while the patient is in labor, it might be possible to perform a postmortem cesarean section in an effort to deliver a living baby.

Some deaths, however, follow a long, low trajectory of the dying process. Time is available for farewells, tying the loose knots, forgiveness, reconciliations, and anticipatory bereavement.

Obstetrics and gynecology is so diverse a field that its boundaries extend from the most limited subspecialization to the most extensive forms of primary care. Too often, doctors overdo specialization. Instead of treating women as persons with fears, worries, and great interest in their disease and its treatment, they take care of only the bleeding fibromyoma. There may be only the briefest contact with the husband and the family, who share the same fears and worries as the patient. Physicians' training, sometimes their temperament, and certainly the times in which they were educated and practice are conducive to this detached approach. The advent of antibiotic drugs 40 years ago changed the medical community from a caring one to a curing one.

Technological advances have pushed physicians closer to the curing side of the health meter and further from the caring side. But the time is long overdue for physicians to leave treatment of symptoms and disease only and to return to treatment of the whole person. They must superimpose psychosocial care on top of the excellent medical care they already give. They must expand to the larger area of concern for the entire person—psyche and soma—who presents only her physical disease for treatment.

Psychiatrists, psychologists, and sociologists have considered what alterations must be made in the physician's role. Cassell (1976) wrote that they must treat the illness beyond the disease. The patient's perception of her disease is the illness; the physician's perception of her illness is the disease.

When doctors read patients' charts or go to morbidity and mortality conferences, they are overwhelmed with laboratory reports, changes in antibiotics, consultation opinions, and so forth. Yet, the patient frequently dies unattended. There is no mention of how she dies or how she was supported. Do nurses' notes and doctors' notes ever report how the patient felt or her psychological reactions to diagnoses, therapy, and the hospital environment and its restrictions?

The plight of a dying pregnant woman is heartrending. The sunshine of one of the brightest events of life is darkened by knowledge of the slow and irreversible process of dying. The young woman worries whether the baby will be mature enough to survive or whether the baby will be affected by her disease, especially if she has cancer. After successful delivery, the patient can be with her baby, although she may not be strong enough to care for it. But her joy is dampened by knowledge of the inexorable nature of her disease and approaching death.

Do health professionals have any meaningful relationships with their dying patients? Shneidman has written the following:

From the psychosocial point of view, the primary task of
helping the dying person is to focus on the person—not on
the biochemistry or pathology of the diseased organs, but
on a human being who is a living beehive of emotions that
include . . . the fight for control and terror. And, with
a dying person, there is another grim, omnipresent fact
in the picture: time is finite. [1977, p. 201]

Obstetrics and gynecology is one of the happiest medical special-
ties. It rarely has to treat the dying patient or deal with death. Neu-
rology, oncology, and cardiology, in contrast, confront fatal illnesses
daily. Feifel (1965) has noted that physicians have chosen their profession as an escape from the fear of death and even from death itself.
It is as though being a member of the healing club will provide protection. If going into medicine is a retreat from death, how much more
so is the selection of gynecology as a specialty? This may explain
the obstetrician/gynecologist's success-cure orientation and the dis-
inclination of some to consider the psychosocial aspects of caring for
the woman who is dying. But the obstetricians and gynecologists are
not alone. Even psychiatrists have the same problem.

Psychiatrists are diffident about treating patients who are
"really sick" unless they also happen to have a readily
identified psychiatric diagnosis. Despite brave words
about the "patient as a whole," psychiatrists who forgo
treating the terminal patient do not understand that their
contribution might be extremely significant in determining whether or not the final hours and days are reason-
ably harmonious. [Weisman 1970, p. 70]

The obstetrician/gynecologist can dispel some fears by telling
the truth to those patients who ask for the facts. It requires the
judgment of Solomon to know how much to tell and when. If the truth
is not told, patients often learn from nonverbal communications
(hemming, changing facial expressions, abrupt departures) or from
a nurse or a resident. The right to know also implies the right not
to know. A small percentage of patients do not want to know, or
deny, the facts after being told. As outlined by Pattison (1977), denial can be existential (the meaning of death), psychological (repression of what is known), nonaccepting (suppression of awareness), and
nonattentive (exclusion of the nondesirable). Pattison has acknowledged the need to respond to a process within care givers and dying
patients that includes both denial and acceptance. Even those who
acknowledge that they are dying have many fears—of the unknown, of
loneliness, of sorrow, of loss of body, of loss of self-control, of
suffering and pain, of loss of identity, and of regression.

Truth telling can be divided into the following categories: who, when, what, how, and where (Finn 1978, p. 172).

Who: The physician is usually the best one to tell the true facts to the patient. However, in circumstances when the patient has been transferred from familiar home surroundings and a doctor whom she knows to the tertiary hospital with superspecialists whom she does not know, the telling may best be done by her family doctor, her husband, her pastor, or a close family friend.

When: Selection of the optimal time is based on judgment supplemented by luck. The optimal time in obstetrics/gynecology is usually soon after surgery or once the patient has passed through the first postsurgical days. Her questions may be indirect and subtle, with many unspoken inferences and a hidden agenda. Overt questions should be answered. If it is felt that enough knowledge has not been imparted, the doctor should ask, "Is there anything else you want to know?" This question may elicit more penetrating queries.

What: What is told should be sufficient to reveal to the patient the diagnosis and the prognosis, as far as they are known. Laypersons' terms should be used. Repetition and rephrasing may be needed. Yet, no other conversation is as meaningful to the patient. This is the only type of talk that serves as a foundation for communication during the entire chronic living-dying phase. If the patient has not been told the truth, the conduct of her care becomes a sham. The obstetrician/gynecologist becomes more deeply immersed in a sea of lies. How can complications or recurrences or new metastases be explained? If the truth has been told once in as complete a fashion as is appropriate, there has been adjustment to the psychological impact of the first telling. The obstetrician/gynecologist builds on the previously established foundation of truth to keep the patient informed. Yet, Weisman has written, "Only in pediatrics and in terminal care is it common practice to tell a patient as little as possible and to ask responsible family members to decide for the patient" (1970, p. 73).

How: The so-called bedside manner is really a projection of physicians themselves—their beliefs, their attitudes, their concerns, their methods of dealing with problems and patients. The how reveals the deepest, inner personality of the obstetrician/gynecologist. Some are gentle, some are brusque, some are evasive, some are forthright to the point of bluntness. Some are fast; some are slow and more inclined to add one chapter at a time until the entire tale has been told.

Where: Usually, this is done in the unsatisfactory environment of a two-bed hospital room with a curious roommate behind the curtain in the other bed. It is better to take the woman to a counseling room, which hospitals rarely provide, or to a treatment room. It is best to talk to the patient in the presence of her husband, so that both will know what has been said and will know that they share this knowledge. This will prevent the closed awareness of the dying patient that some families wish to enforce on the terminal situation: "You know that I am dying, I know that you know, but we cannot let each other know." After I have spoken with a patient, I write in the chart what I have said and ask the charge nurse to incorporate it in her report so that all staff members will know.

There appears to be a singular inappropriateness when the patient is a young woman who is pregnant or who has recently given birth. She has lived so short a time. She has had extensive surgery, perhaps irradiation, and now chemotherapy. Despite all that has been done, her prospects are dim. The savage unfairness shakes the nurses who empathize more with her than with older patients. Many nurses and doctors need a support system after such repetitious encounters day after day. Kastenbaum suggested that

> the staff's anguish often remains "illegitimate." They are
> not supposed to be suffering. They do not have the "right"
> to suffer in the same way as terminally ill patients and
> their families do. [1977, p. 233]

Because little of their training and experience prepares professionals for the distress they feel in caring for the terminally ill, the phenomenon of staff suffering is not openly expressed or acknowledged, which makes it even more difficult to bear. When staff seek to stay in control, then it is not only a matter of controlling what is outside (the patient's situation) but also what is inside (the staff members' emotions).

Finally, the psychosocial transition time occurs. Opportunities for curing are long gone. Active therapy is now displaced by caring. The terminal phase provides opportunity for the obstetrician/gynecologist to give the best psychosocial care to the patient. The doctor visits frequently, even at odd times—for example, while waiting for an operating room—to sit down with the patient, to hold her hand, to listen. Medication to relieve pain will be prescribed as it is needed. Hospital administrators will be urged to be flexible on policies concerning visitors, food, and extra attentions. Thus, the last phase of living can be faced with courage, perception, resolution, individuality, and appropriateness.

> Physicians are prone to a kind of professional as well as
> personal despair. Death is always their enemy, but death
> cannot be defeated. The doctor may win a skirmish, even

a battle, but sooner or later the struggle is over and his capitulation is ensured. In some instances, the incentive to care for a terminal patient may wane as cure becomes more remote. Yet, the solitude of dying and the dilemma of a conscientious physician can be relieved somewhat by paying closer attention to the agonies within the social field in which death occurs. It cannot be claimed that attention to psychosocial factors will extend life, even for an hour. There is evidence, however, that physicians, including psychiatrists, can help to prevent lonely and anguished deaths. . . . To do so, the doctor must be accessible as a person, not only available as a physician. He can then maintain respect for the patient because his primary antipathy will be directed only toward the cause of suffering, not toward the person who suffers, whether that person is the patient or the doctor himself. [Weisman 1970, p. 75]

Although most dying occurs in the hospital, this is not necessary. The terminal event, death, may have to take place in a hospital because the patient is comatose, is incontinent of urine and feces, is in intractable pain, or has lost cortical brain function. But the process of dying, the so-called living-dying phase, can occur at home or in a day hospital (where patients go home at night) or in a hospice. The physical and mental condition of the patient, the facilities in her home, the resources available in the community, and the attitude of the spouse and family are the chief determinants of the best location for the dying process.

Shneidman has written the following:

I believe that every physician should be a clinical thanatologist at least once (preferably early) in his or her career, and thus deal intensively (5 or 6 days a week, for an hour each day) with the personal-human-psychological aspects of a dying person.

This means sitting unhurriedly by the bedside and coming to know that dying person qua dying person—over and above the biochemistry, cytology, medicine, and oncology of the case. This also means not avoiding the dying and death aspects of the situation, but learning about them, sharing them, being burdened by them (and their enormous implications)—in short, sharing the intensity of the thanatological experience. [1977, p. 210]

Philosophers, sociologists, social workers, psychologists, and chaplains have censured physicians for not giving adequate and appropriate care to patients who are in the process of dying. These criticisms may be deserved, for care given at this time probably is not as good as the care given to an acutely ill patient who will recover. Physicians have abdicated their role to other specialists. However, obstetricians and gynecologists have a unique role to act as caring human beings with special technical knowledge of the diseases they are treating.

REFERENCES

American Medical Association. 1964. Guide for Maternal Death Studies. Chicago: American Medical Association.

Cassell, E. J. 1976. The Healer's Art. Philadelphia: J. B. Lippincott.

Feifel, H. 1965. "The Function of Attitudes towards Death." In Death and Dying: Attitudes of Patient and Doctor, pp. 633-41. New York: Group for the Advancement of Psychiatry.

Finn, W. F. 1978. "Will Your Doctor Tell You That You Are Dying and Do You Really Want to Know?" In The Dying Human, edited by A. DeVries and A. Carni, pp. 171-81. Tel Aviv, Israel: Turtle Dove Publishing.

Kastenbaum, R. 1977. "In Control." In Psychosocial Care of the Dying Patient, edited by C. A. Garfield, pp. 227-40. New York: McGraw-Hill.

Pattison, E. M. 1977. "The Living-Dying Process." In Psychosocial Care of the Dying Patient, edited by C. A. Garfield, pp. 133-68. New York: McGraw-Hill.

Shneidman, E. S. 1977. "Some Aspects of Psychotherapy with Dying Patients." In Psychosocial Care of the Dying Patient, edited by C. A. Garfield, pp. 201-26. New York: McGraw-Hill.

Weisman, A. D. 1970. "Misgivings and Misconception in the Psychiatric Care of Terminal Patients." Psychiatry 33(1):67-81.

18
Implications of Ovarian Cancer

Yvonne M. Parnes

Ovarian cancer has to be the best-kept gynecologic secret! Generally, women are oblivious to it. This author has questioned women in many walks of life, some medically oriented and some not. Few, if any, knew of the devastation that ovarian cancer brings and the catastrophic illness it is. The disease is a medical and surgical nightmare, and it leads to death.

With the emergence of the women's movement, male gynecologists were forced to retrench to consider patients' expectations of them and their attitudes toward women. Nothing has come forth from such introspection to better the tragic plight of those who are fatally ill with ovarian cancer. While arguments persist as to the best way to treat breast cancer and while women are making decisions that they often are not prepared to make, except in fear, the advances in treating ovarian cancer are few. Breast cancer patients have a good chance of survival. Ovarian cancer patients can be virtually helpless in their bout with a familial disease that threatens female offspring.

Most women have no information about ovarian cancer. They are unfamiliar with the destructiveness of the disease and the inability of modern technology to detect it in an early stage. Yet, ovarian can-

The author wishes to acknowledge the opportunity for her collaboration with the "I Can Cope" program, sponsored by the Queens and Long Island chapters of the American Cancer Society; the knowledge imparted by the conferences of the department of obstetrics/gynecology of Long Island Jewish-Hillside Medical Center, New Hyde Park, New York, and Dr. Joseph Rovinsky, chairperson; Dr. Burton Krumholz, chairman, Queens Hospital Center, Long Island Jewish affiliation, for his personal communications with her on oophorectomy and hysterectomy; and the ovarian cancer patients of the Community Health Program of Nassau County, who have communicated bravery and sincerity.

cer accounts for more deaths than any other gynecologic cancer. More controversies surround the treatment of ovarian cancer than any other gynecologic cancer. Insidious, silent, fatal—ovarian cancer defies us and eludes the edict that early detection can cure. There is no method of early diagnosis. Nor does it respect age: it attacks late teenagers, women through the childbearing years, and postmenopausal women who thought that any disease of the reproductive organs was limited to the menstrual years. The warning signs of cancer have become familiar reading in public places, buses, subways, on television, in the newspapers, and in magazines, but they offer no hint of anything associated with ovarian disease. There seem to be no early signs, no detectable symptoms to give a warning.

Patients come to experts who treat diseases that affect only women, secure that we will give our best to do our best for them. We become more human, less omnipotent, when we admit that we have no solutions. There is much that we do not know about ovarian disease and little to offer once it is established. Paternalism in medicine often obscures reality. To protect patients instead of educating them is to play ostrich. It is sobering for physicians to be confronted with patients with ovarian cancer. They must summon all their compassion and knowledge to forget the possibility that it may be something they alone can treat. The abilities of many experts are required to guide these patients and their families to an understanding of the enormous problems, with hope ever present and care givers always available. It must be demonstrated that we need to reach out into the community to learn what is new and to find a suitable volunteer to lead the patient in her course of treatment, as perhaps that volunteer was led. Knowing someone with a similar diagnosis and hearing from that person what it is to go through the surgery, chemotherapy, and even a "second look" operation gives the patient an informed and supportive hand to hold.

THE FAMILY

The family of the woman with ovarian cancer becomes unusually stressed and thanatologically involved. A huge toll is extracted from all, because the disease is visibly debilitating and costly, possibly with periods of supposed remission followed by devastation. Female family members often develop symptoms similar to those of the sick relative. If the family will permit truths, ongoing counseling of the entire family may be meaningful. It can help to prepare for support at home, if this is possible, and eliminate much guilt in the future. There must be an acceptance of responsibility. The American Cancer Society has an "I Can Cope" program, an eight-week course for the patient and significant others. It is an educational, informative course that offers some understanding of what has occurred and what resources are available. It augments with literature, experts in nutrition, exercise, psychotherapy, pain therapy, estate planning, and open talk. It touches on areas of illness previously misunderstood by patients and families. It brings some order to the chaos created by sudden diagnosis and rapid change from well person to sick and/or dying patient. It organizes a network of care givers when families feel alone and intimidated by disease and despair.

It is suggested that the physician initiate a discussion with female family members to alert them to the often-familial tendencies of this disease. As noted above, even with sophisticated screening technology we still cannot detect its presence early. Preventive measures can include a prophylactic oophorectomy at the end of the childbearing years. The likelihood that a woman in a high risk family will develop ovarian cancer is 17 times greater than in the general population. In the author's own patient population, there have been seven instances involving maternal grandmother, mother, and daughter. Although it is perhaps a disturbing consideration, prophylactic surgery offers the only way to control familial ovarian cancer.

Gynecologists have to recognize the thanatologic implications for the family with ovarian disease. They must institute careful surveillance of these potentially involved patients and educate them to the risk factors. Early gastric symptoms should be carefully investigated, and counseling by the gynecologist and another expert equipped to give a second opinion can guide the patient appropriately.

PREVENTION

During the annual or semiannual pelvic examination, the ovaries must be carefully assessed. A rectovaginal examination should be performed to examine the ovaries properly. Should there be any question about the size of the ovaries, sonographic examination may be employed to attempt to rule out early changes or disease.

Prior to a hysterectomy, the question of whether or not to remove the ovaries always arises. Women rely on the judgment of their physician to do what is best. Women must be counseled and encouraged to participate in the decision making without making decisions that they are not prepared to make. It is perilous to fail to consider carefully leaving ovaries after hysterectomy. Family history must be explored for ovarian disease not previously identified. Proximity to menopause should be cited, and the efficiency of estrogen replacement therapy in avoiding menopausal symptoms and osteoporosis should be stressed. Controversy over estrogen therapy has confused many women and the thought of taking oral estrogen is frightening. However, survival of the patient should be the primary consideration.

CHEMOTHERAPY

The chemotherapy following cytoreductive surgery for ovarian cancer is strenuous. It is a costly, exhausting, nightmarish confrontation with panic because it is a gamble and reduces one to measuring time. It captures the weak, challenges the strong, and enlists the patient in a struggle. It can make time stand still. It can offer hope to those who cherish life enough to fight beyond all comprehension for whatever it can achieve. It can make the patient an invalid and involve the family in supportive care giving. Many patients have stopped treatment, preferring death to nausea, weakness, inability to eat or drink, and the requirement of constant care. Each individual has the right to determine if she can go on. There are no medals for such valor and often there is great physical and emotional pain.

After the initial course of chemotherapy, there is no peace; there is another surgical bout called second look.

SECOND LOOK OPERATION

This hurdle is for women who have undergone appropriate initial surgery followed by chemotherapy for a specific time and who then show no clinical, radiological, or other evidence of persistent cancer. Residual disease has been discovered in 36 percent of patients undergoing the second operation. This surgery is performed to restage the extent of the disease and to plan further therapy or to confirm a lack of clinical response to first-line chemotherapy. The patient must be persuaded to undergo another procedure to make certain that her success is real. There are false-negative rates in other modes of assessing disease status and the potential good far outweighs the inconvenience and the expense, say the surgeons. The procedure is extensive and requires the skills of the most meticulous gynecologic oncologist. The incision extends from the symphysis to eight centimeters above the umbilicus. That alone tells the patient the magnitude of this disease. The risks of anesthesia, the length of recuperation, the second confrontation with hope and doubt can severely damage the patient's chances of ever leaving the protective custody of her doctors. She has the right to know what is in store for her. Few patients ask because they are so involved in trying to face each day, dependent on family to provide and care for them. They may survive for a time and suffer. Two-thirds of the patients will have complications after surgery, such as hemorrhage, fistula, or renal failure.

It may also mean economic exhaustion for a family. The advantages and risks should be clearly defined—but rarely are. The patient is usually a pawn in a study, a number in a protocol, a statistic. The average family knows little of this, perhaps thinking that what they have seen and heard on television is a figment of someone's imagination and "cannot happen here." Anger mounts as they proceed from procedure to treatment and back to procedure without any guarantee. Years may go by in a fight that cannot be won. Where honesty, empathy, and respect are needed, only guilt and isolation can be anticipated when the questions asked have no answers. Maintaining quality in the patient's life is, perhaps, the only resolution for the dilemma imposed by aggressive treatment.

RADIATION THERAPY

Radiation therapy is as good as any drug used for ovarian cancer. However, the field to be radiated is so extensive that radiation sickness is almost as difficult to cope with as the reactions from chemotherapy. Whole abdominal radiation and concurrent chemotherapy appear to offer encouraging results. At the moment, the best we can hope for is prolonged survival.

NURSING

Nursing care for this patient presents an enormous challenge to even the most dedicated, skilled, and caring of nurses. The care plan provides an opportunity to nurture, soothe, tend, support, and give quality care to another woman. It is a demanding task that requires sincerity and the ability to listen and to deal in truths. Physical comfort alone is not the only aim of supplication; perception must be used to anticipate the pitfalls that this illness can create.

Initially, a tentative bond can be established between patient and care giver; this is reinforced with great trust at each subsequent encounter. The patient has to know that she can depend on the nurse to support her through all the doubt and pain that come from fighting the illness. She will need positive encouragement and honest warmth when others may turn from the responsibility of caring enough and giving enough.

With alteration in body image and the associated embarrassment that may accompany chemotherapy, expressions of love and caring are important. A flattering scarf or turban, if a wig cannot be worn in bed, gives color to a face puffed by steroids and shields a head showing alopecia. Meticulous hygiene eliminates odors that the patient may notice. Frequent and thorough mouth care, particularly after meals, prevents stomatitis. Turning and passive exercise prevent decubiti and possible contractures and help to keep muscles toned. A walker can be used because ambulatory patients show a marked difference in response to therapies. Fluids and bulk in the diet must be kept in mind, especially when anorexia is present.

There cannot be social isolation for patients. Mental stimulation is provided in the form of visitation, reading, and television viewing. Adding flowers or a taste treat to the tray provides something worth looking forward to when the appetite is poor. The activities of daily living must be preserved until it is necessary to offer total care for the patient's every need. At that time, it is hoped that terminal care can be accomplished in the home with input from a hospice team. Family members can alternate with nurses so that no one person is emotionally exhausted.

The chemotherapy room in the outpatient setting should be cheerful looking, comfortably warm but not oppressive, with music or even a television set available to detract from the tedious treatment. Nausea should be anticipated and preliminary oral antiemetics and easy-to-administer suppositories should be available. Marihuana, either in cigarettes or as tetrahydrocannabinol capsules, may be tried to control nausea. Sucking an ice pop gives sugar and fluid while keeping the mouth moist.

Pain management requires expert prescribing for the multiple kinds of pain that metastatic disease produces. This has become a specialty. The armamentarium includes drugs that give a sense of well-being concurrent with pain control.

Throughout the time the nurse is associated with the patient and family, the opportunity to educate endures. It is in the nurse's realm to provide answers to patients and families when physicians are not available. The nurse must be cautious to teach without imparting her own values or biases. In this disease, because so little is known and the aggressive measures used to treat it so debilitating, the nurse must discreetly balance support and uncertainty. Each patient may be seen as a step to significant success in eventually making some progress in either detection or eradication of ovarian cancer. Despite personal identification with patients, nurses must remember that they are one of a chain on the professional team. They cannot assume full control, except to do their work with the utmost compassion for the good of the patient and the family.

CONCLUSION

Women should concern themselves with their major health issues and not rely on the medical establishment alone for education about their own bodies. They must be aware of all issues that threaten their right to make decisions for themselves. Women have to provoke the medical community to think in terms of disease prevention as well as disease treatment. In ovarian cancer, the only answer at present for those in the high risk category is prophylactic intervention.

No woman should ever have to say, "I didn't know" about anything that pertains to her own well-being. It is her duty to know as much about herself as she can learn in an effort to prevent death from a disease that cannot be detected until it is too late. We all deserve the best that modern medical knowledge can give us. We need to be prepared for every eventuality that can occur—even for the silent killers.

19

Gynecologic Cancer: Stages of Illness and Therapy

Vincent Vinciguerra

A full spectrum of problems are encountered in the treatment of women with gynecologic cancer. On the one hand, we can offer effective, curative treatment to many patients so afflicted. On the other hand, treatment is rendered to patients who will eventually die from cancer, although they initially present with treatable disease. Many of the principles of treatment utilized for the care of these patients are applicable to other types of malignancies.

The most common types of gynecologic malignancies include cervical, uterine, and ovarian cancer (Weiss, Homochuk, and Young 1977). Cancer of the vulva, vagina, and uterine tubes is very rare (Lingeman 1974). As a result of early diagnosis, the incidence of cancer of the cervix has markedly decreased in frequency since 1947 (Conroy et al. 1976). However, uterine and ovarian cancers have been increasing in frequency.

The patient's initial conflict occurs at the time of the first visit to the physician. An examination is performed, and the patient is told that an abdominal mass is present. This can be called the issue of discovery. Ovarian cancer is an insidious disease because (1) the patient often presents with widespread cancer by the time symptoms begin or (2) the presence of disease is discovered on routine examination. Many questions go through the patient's mind at this time: "How could this happen?" "Is the correct diagnosis being made?" "Did I do anything wrong?" "Should I go for a second opinion?" Some patients had had examinations six or twelve months earlier and had been told that everything was normal.

The next phase in treating the illness can be called the issue of full knowledge. Arrangements for admission to the hospital should be made quickly in order to minimize the anxiety of waiting for something to be done. One quick sweep of the surgeon's scalpel and the

141

diagnosis is made. With ovarian cancer, diagnosis and initial treatment are performed simultaneously. The first principle of treatment (besides taking a biopsy) is to remove as much of the tumor as possible and, hopefully, debulk and leave the patient with minimal residual cancer. The ultimate prognosis is determined by the stage of the disease, or how advanced the cancer is. For patients in the earliest stage, the two-year survival rate is 80 percent and the five-year survival rate is 70 percent (Yoonessi and Hresh Chy Shyn 1978). Patients with more advanced disease, however, have a 5-to-10 percent survival rate. Unfortunately, when the diagnosis of ovarian cancer is made, 70 percent of patients have stage 3 or 4 disease, which represents cancer that surgery alone cannot cure. Removing as much tumor as possible allows chemotherapy to be more effective and results in higher complete remissions and cures (Ozols et al. 1981).

The phase that now confronts the patient is the issue of decision. The patient is told the diagnosis and the extensiveness of the cancer. She is told that chemotherapy will be required as an important step in attempting to cure the disease. This is a particularly difficult issue for patients because they have only recently recovered from extensive surgery and have been told that their cancer has been removed or that there are only minimal residual cancer cells present. They are just getting back on their feet and returning to normal patterns of nutrition. Now we tell them we are going to treat them with chemicals that will make them sick again.

In order to appreciate the turmoil that these patients will face, it is important to understand the results of chemotherapy for ovarian cancer. Five to ten years ago, many patients received chemotherapeutic agents that were nontoxic. Recommending chemotherapy for ovarian cancer patients was not difficult. The results were not good, however, as the chance of obtaining complete remissions was only 10 to 15 percent (Tobias and Griffitles 1976). Since then, we have developed more aggressive combination chemotherapy programs, including drugs such as cyclophosphamide, adriamycin, and Cisplatinum. These drugs are combined to form a highly toxic program, which is also highly effective. Complete remission rates have now increased to between 50 and 80 percent, and the potential for cure ranges between 40 to 60 percent of patients (Vogl et al. 1981).

The toxic side effects, however, have increased significantly. The major ill effects of the combination chemotherapy program include nausea and vomiting. Platinum is an extremely toxic drug that can cause severe vomiting that lasts hours or sometimes days with certain patients. The drugs to control vomiting and nausea are not always effective. Over 20 such drugs are commonly used, including Compazine, marihuana or tetrahydrocannabinol, or even tranquilizers (Frytak and Moertel 1981). More recently, a new drug, reglan (metoclopramide), has brought increased control of vomiting (Strum et al. 1982). Besides the vomiting from the chemotherapy itself, which occurs several hours after receiving the drug, another common issue in these patients is the complication of anticipatory vomiting (Morrow and Morrell 1982). It begins prior to treatment as soon as the patient approaches the hospital and the doctor's office. Vomiting starts as a reflex before the chemotherapy is given. In an attempt to control this difficult reaction, psychiatrists and social workers are studying the use of hypnosis for such patients.

Besides vomiting, patients are at risk to develop kidney failure and suppression of blood counts (Prestayko, D'Aoust, and Crooke 1979). This can result in increased susceptibility to infection. Another psychologically important side effect of chemotherapy is hair loss. This effect can significantly alter body image, yet most patients accept the complications and agree to chemotherapy. The patients require a great deal of physical and psychological support, not only from members of the hospital staff but also from family members. The primary goal of chemotherapy is not only to increase the number of complete remissions but also to maintain the complete remissions for long durations, ultimately resulting in cures. Currently, our drugs are more effective but have increased side effects that the patients must endure.

In order to prevent recurrence of disease, treatment must be given over a prolonged period of time, lasting nine to twelve months. After chemotherapy is completed, the patient is advised that further evaluation is necessary. The only certain way to guarantee that there is no residual cancer is to perform another operation, the "second-look" procedure (Wilson et al. 1981). It is our practice to present this to the patient at the beginning of treatment, so that she understands that it will not be a sudden decision to undergo further surgery. Although sophisticated diagnostic techniques are available (sonograms, X rays, and CAT scans of the abdomen), these tests are notoriously inaccurate in predicting relapse from treatment. Most patients will accept further surgery even though they have suffered a great deal of toxicity from the chemotherapy. A few patients either have refused chemotherapy after three or four cycles or have refused the second look procedure, feeling that everything has been done for them.

Some patients' disease no longer responds to treatment; it is incurable. These are not only patients with ovarian cancer but also patients with other types of malignancies. Treatment is still offered but is intended to result in the control of symptoms, or palliation; it is not aimed to cure.

In 1979 North Shore University Hospital in Manhasset, New York, started the Don Monti Home Oncology Medical Extension (HOME) program (Vinceguerra et al. 1980, 1983). This is a special program for nonambulatory cancer patients whose alternative for treatment would be hospitalization. Patients are given the option to remain at home, where they can receive palliative and supportive care in the presence of their families. A van was purchased and equipped with medical machines to help perform blood tests and to allow administration of chemotherapy at home. The patient population is contained with a ten-mile radius, which allows for sufficient follow-up care. A multi-specialty team is transported on the van to the home. The team includes oncologists, oncology nurses, social workers, a nutritionist, a medical technologist, and consultant staff.

Eligibility criteria for this program include a histologic diagnosis of cancer, affiliation with a doctor on the hospital's staff, residence within the ten-mile radius, and most important, willingness on the part of the family and the patient to receive home care. The HOME program is part of a hospice program that is home-based and utilizes the hospital for backup treatment in extreme emergencies. The median age of patients is 62. The average survival is slightly more than two months. Only 30 percent of patients are receiving active anticancer treatment and transfusions. Most patients receive only supportive care—pain control, nutritional support, and psychosocial counseling. At least one-half of the patients are allowed to remain at home to die. This is in contrast to data derived from the New York State Department of Health, which indicate that only 15 to 20 percent of patients living in Nassau and Suffolk counties die at home without intensive home support. Most patients throughout the country are dying in hospitals or in nursing home facilities.

The HOME program has been found to be highly successful and greatly appreciated by the patients and their families (Vinciguerra et al. 1983). Patients are allowed to decide what type of treatment will be received and the location where it will be given. Dignity and self-respect can be maintained. Besides the psychological benefits of home treatment, the care-giving team has found that nutritional support, pain control, survival, and cost benefit are superior for patients treated at home compared with hospitalized, terminal cancer patients.

In surveying the impact of gynecologic cancer, one can start with the presupposition of impending doom and loss. Perhaps more emphasis should be placed on the potential for gain. It is possible for patients to gain from health professionals who are able to render advice and improved treatments. Patients can also gain by getting to know themselves better as they encounter life crises and attempt to conquer life-threatening illness. Medical professionals themselves can gain knowledge and sensitivity as they listen to patients and try to offer them the best care possible.

REFERENCES

Conroy, J. F., G. C. Lewis, L. Brady et al. 1976. "Low Dose Bleomycin in Cervical Cancer." Cancer 37: 660.

Frytak, S., and C. G. Moertel. 1981. "Management of Nausea and Vomiting in the Cancer Patient." Journal of the American Medical Association 245: 393.

Lingeman, C. H. 1974. "Etiology of Cancer of the Ovary." Journal of the National Cancer Institute 53: 1603.

Morrow, G. R., and C. Morell. 1982. "Behavioral Treatment for Anticipatory Nausea and Vomiting Induced by Cancer Chemotherapy." New England Journal of Medicine 307: 1476.

Ozols, R. F., R. I. Fisher, T. Anderson et al. 1981. "Peritoneoscopy in the Management of Ovarian Cancer." American Journal of Obstetrics and Gynecology 140: 611.

Prestayko, A. W., J. C. D'Aoust, and S. T. Crooke. 1979. "Cisplatinum." Cancer Treatment Review 6: 17.

Strum, S. B., J. E. McDermed, R. W. Opfell, and C. P. Prech. 1982. "Intravenous Metoclopramide." Journal of the American Medical Association 247: 2683.

Tobias, J. S., and C. T. Griffitles. 1976. "Management of Ovarian Carcinoma." New England Journal of Medicine 294: 877.

Vinciguerra, V. P., T. Degnan, J. Diener et al. 1980. "Home Oncology Medical Extension. A New Home Treatment Program." CA—A Cancer Journal for Clinicians 30: 182.

Vinciguerra, V. P., T. Degnan, M. O'Connell et al. 1983. "Bringing Terminal Care Home. An Effective Program." Your Patient and Cancer 187.

Vogl, S., M. Berenzweig, B. Kaplan et al. 1981. "The CHAD and the HAD Regimen in Ovarian Cancer." Cancer Treatment Reports 63: 311.

Weiss, N. S., T. Homochuk, and J. C. Young. 1977. "Incidence of Histologic Types of Ovarian Cancer." Gynecologic Oncology 5: 161.

Wilson, J. K., R. F. Ozols, B. Lewis, and R. C. Young. 1981. "Current Status of Therapeutic Modalities for Treatment of Gynecologic Malignancies." American Journal of Obstetrics and Gynecology 141: 91.

Yoonessi, M., and M. Hresh Chy Shyn. 1978. "Surgical Staging of Gynecologic Cancer." New York State Journal of Medicine, November, p. 2030.

20

Home Oncology Medical Extension

Arlene Sciortino

The Home Oncology Medical Extension (HOME) van of North Shore University Hospital, Manhasset, New York, attempts to provide services to meet patients' needs on an individual basis. Most of the services are directed toward comfort, symptom relief, and education of family members. Physical examinations are done by the physician and the oncology nurse. The nurse visits the patient weekly or on an as-needed basis for the evaluation of symptoms and the appropriate adjustment of medications. Visits by the physician are usually monthly, or they can be scheduled when a situation arises necessitating a major change in treatment plan or when the physician's presence will lend additional emotional support to the patient and family.

Patient and family teaching is ongoing, and wherever possible, the family is supported as the primary provider of care for the patient. Psychosocial support is provided by the team's social worker, who visits all patients. Social worker visits may also be scheduled apart from the medical team whenever necessary or as a follow-up to the van team visit. It is our experience that the entire team contributes in a significant way to the support of the patient and family.

For selected patients, active chemotherapy treatment is available. Blood transfusions are utilized in conjunction with chemotherapy when indicated. Transfusions are also provided in cases where the transfusion will offer additional physical support and symptom palliation, as in severe dyspnea or weakness associated with alterations in blood status. Nutrition education is provided by the oncology dietitian, who also visits all the patients with the team. Specific problems can be addressed on an individual basis, and tube feedings are utilized based on an assessment by a medical team. Bereavement care is offered on a group or individual basis when necessary, and all families are contacted by the staff at least once by home visit or telephone during the immediate bereavement period.

To illustrate how the program works and how the services are actually utilized, a case study of a patient who was treated on the HOME van follows.

Mrs. S, aged 32 years, was married, the mother of a three-year-old boy, and at the time of the diagnosis, eight months pregnant. The patient was admitted to the hospital on July 31, 1981. For several months prior to admission, Mrs. S had complained of severe pain on the left side and back. The pain was aching and constant and had increased in intensity. She had also been complaining of constipation. A sonogram revealed a single intrauterine fetus in a cephalic presentation. The gestational age was approximated at 36 weeks. Fetal heartbeat was noted to be normal and what was seen as the fetus likewise was within normal limits. The patient's abdomen was scanned and marked and bilateral hydronephrosis was seen. This hydronephrosis was greater than one would expect in a simple pregnancy. In addition, multiple masses were noted. The palpable mass in the left lower quadrant was seen to be composed of solid tissue with necrosis within it. Most of the other masses were within the liver. These findings were characteristic of metastatic cancer. The patient was then admitted to the hospital.

Review of systems revealed a history of weight loss of more than ten pounds in the last few months. Total weight gain in pregnancy was nine pounds. There was a history of recent anorexia, fatigue and tiredness, and difficulty sleeping. There was also a history of a dry cough in the last few weeks. Past medical history revealed no diabetes; no hypertension; no tuberculosis; no cardiac, kidney, or pulmonary disorders. Psychosocial history was likewise negative. The patient was allergic to penicillin.

Gynecologic history: The patient began menstruating at the age of 13. Her periods occurred every 28 to 30 days and lasted five days. The patient had no dysmenorrhea.

Obstetrical history: The patient had one spontaneous normal delivery in July of 1978. There were no previous gynecologic problems.

Social history: Mrs. S smoked two packs of cigarettes per day for eight years and stopped in midpregnancy. She did not drink.

Family history: Her father died at age 52 of a massive stroke, her mother at age 47 of heart disease. Maternal grandmother died at age 59 of breast cancer. Sister and brother both have hypertension but are alive and well.

On physical examination, Mrs. S presented as an emaciated female who appeared to be in no acute distress. Her vital signs were normal. Examination of the head and neck were negative. Her lungs were clear and heart sounds normal. Abdomen revealed a gravid uterus, the size of which was difficult to evaluate. There was a mass on the left side below the costal margin that was soft and tender. No lymph nodes were palpated. The impression of the admitting doctor was that there was an abdominal mass and that widespread malignancy would have to be ruled out. The patient's admitting orders included weight every day, diet as tolerated, blood work and chest X ray, intravenous therapy, monitoring of fetal heart rate, and pain medication. After consultation with the obstetrician, it was decided that a laparotomy would be done to deliver the fetus and examine the abdomen. Prior to surgery the patient was transfused. On August 5, 1981, the patient was taken to the operating room, and an exploratory laparotomy was performed. A healthy infant girl, five pounds, ten ounces, was delivered via a cesarean section. At the time of inspection, the abdomen was seen to contain multiple tumor nodules. One large section almost completely obliterated the right kidney. The tumor was presumed to have originated in the uterus in its first route and then metastasized to the abdomen as well as to the liver. Biopsy was done and the patient was closed. Results of the biopsy revealed leiomyosarcoma, the tumor arising from smooth muscles and underlying connective tissue.

On August 10, 1981, the patient was seen by the medical oncologist, who suggested chemotherapy after the patient recovered from surgery. Her postoperative course was uneventful and the patient was discharged from the hospital one week later. The patient was subsequently treated in the oncology department for chemotherapy and pain control. She was readmitted to the hospital on October 29, 1981, complaining of increased weakness and pain. The feeling at this time was that she had failed the chemotherapy regime and that the goal of therapy now would be comfort, nutrition, pain control, and general supportive care. This was ordered in the hospital; the patient was discharged in November. Mrs. S was then picked up by the HOME van.

At this time, she was extremely cachectic, confined to bed, alert and oriented, but very weak. Her main complaints were pain and nausea. A regime of pain medications was instituted and an abdominal X ray ordered to be done at home to assess whether intestinal obstruction was present. Two days later, a second visit was made to assess the efficacy of the pain medications. X ray revealed intestinal obstruction and the patient refused hospitalization. At this juncture, Mrs. S was on home care from the hospital and had a hospital bed and a home health aide four hours a day. The visiting nurse came in once a week.

The doctor saw the patient at home on November 10. Mr. S was caring for his wife while his parents looked after the three-year-old boy and the infant. On November 16, Mrs. S was still awake and alert. The last visit to the patient was made on November 23. On November 24, 1981, the patient expired at home.

The support system for this patient had included her family. The husband was the primary care giver, while the mother-in-law took over child care. While the patient was able, she had tried to care for her infant, but within a short time this became too difficult. She felt resentful because she had to relinquish control of her children to her mother-in-law, but she realized that she was not physically able to care for them. The visiting nurse came to the patient's home twice a week for evaluation and ongoing physical and emotional support. Volunteers were provided to sit with the patient in order to give the husband a respite from constant attendance. Finally, the HOME van provided supportive care with visits from the physician, the nurse oncologist, dietitian, medical technologist, and social worker. Psychosocial support and counseling were available to the patient and family members.

The care accorded this patient and her family enabled her to die at home with a minimum of suffering and with the feeling that neither she nor her family had been abandoned. More important, she remained in both spirit and mind a viable member of her family until her death.

21

Ethical Tension: Casework and Psychosocial Research with the Terminally Ill

Denis C. Carlton

Psychosocial research and psychosocial support for patients, with shared concomitant elements of design and implementation, have been basic tenets of the Don Monti Home Oncology Medical Extension (HOME) program. In the original National Cancer Institute grant that funded the program, the protocol called for administration of psychosocial trait measures over an extended evaluation period (Vinciguerra et al. 1980). It was postulated that patients receiving the supportive services of program staff in their own homes would demonstrate less anxiety and depression, enhanced coping skills, and a higher degree of family equilibrium.

The Profile of Mood States (POMS) and the Multiple Affective Adjective Check List (MAACL) were to be given to patients both at home and in hospital at the time of initial interview, on succeeding weeks for the first month, and then on succeeding months for a total testing period of six months. A separate measure, the Moos Family Environment Scale, was also to be administered to both patient and family during the patient's third week on the study. Responsibility for securing these data, according to the prescribed protocol, was placed with project social work staff.

Apart from the psychosocial research, the social work staff were also charged with the responsibility of performing their more traditional roles with patients and their families. Toward this end, each worker's initial and ongoing obligation was to assess the patient, her family, and her environment. Through assessment, individualized treatment plans emerged. The provision of psychosocial support varied from the simple presence of the social worker with a patient to the delicate and sensitized role of helping the patient and family to communicate with one another or with staff.   Often, this communication was the prime issue with our patients. Where indicated, the social worker encouraged patients and families to verbalize their feelings. A sense of powerlessness, helplessness, or hopelessness all too often combined to promote a self-definition of impotence and lowered self-esteem. Feelings of anticipatory grief and mourning, isolation and abandonment, and guilt and anger were frequently identified as stumbling blocks to continued family functioning. New responsibilities, reversals of roles, and a marked decrease in time available for outside and personal pursuits constituted added burdens that posed threats to positive, adaptive family functioning.

By attempting to share some of the responsibility with families through regular home visiting, the social workers endeavored to establish limits on individual responsibilities. Encouraging and supporting family members to maintain their role functioning and to respect the patient's need for exercising as much control as possible, the workers sought to promote and preserve an equilibrium for the family. Through regular, positive feedback to both patient and family, staff endeavored to reduce the emotional overload and degree of stress. These activities were all in keeping with the avowed goal of maintaining patients in the community by providing and maximizing the psychosocial support they required.

Following an initial collation of research data, several significant questions concerning the original research design confronted those who were involved in the HOME program. The case of Mrs. S (see Chapter 20) is illustrative of such findings.

To recapitulate, Mrs. S was a married 32-year-old woman with one child who was diagnosed as having metastatic cancer during her eighth month of pregnancy. Following a cesarean delivery, she was found to have widespread disease throughout her abdomen, and a definitive diagnosis of leiomyosarcoma was made. After readmission, she was eventually discharged home with the goals of comfort, pain control, and supportive care. The social worker assigned to the research study was to begin the testing protocol with this alert and oriented—but extremely weak—patient.

While protocol called for the administration of both the POMS and MAACL tests weekly, the worker noted the patient's need for caring for her family, relating with her husband, and planning for their future. Acknowledging the patient's diminished endurance and seeking to magnify her comfort, the worker chose instead to use her time with the patient for supportive counseling. No psychosocial testing was ever done with Mrs. S.

While this is a graphic depiction of the conflict inherent in the duality of the social worker's role expectations, it was by no means a unique phenomenon. Of an initial 104 study patients, 83 like Mrs. S had been deemed fit for assessment (Vinciguerra et al. 1984). Of these 83 patients, 60 had completed one POMS test and 32 had completed two or more POMS assessments. Of all 104 patients, only 40 had completed more than one-half of all tests dictated by study protocol (Vinciguerra et al. 1984). In effect, it was discovered that an adequate sample could not be secured from which to begin statistical evaluation.

The primary reason for this noncompliance was that for 37 percent of the scheduled test dates, workers found that the patient's medical and/or physical state precluded the possibility of actual testing (Vinciguerra et al. 1984). The patient's mental and/or emotional state (with problems such as confusion, anxiety, and depression) accounted for an additional 15 percent of noncompliance. Other factors beyond the control of the patient such as language barriers, educational deficits, visitors, and the like constituted another 15 percent. Finally, all other unknown factors made up the remaining 33 percent of noncompliance.

The underlying issue for noncompliance, which was of strategic importance for the study, became apparent through discussion with project social work staff. That issue was the difficulty engendered in having social work staff perform both the role of psychosocial researcher and the role of psychosocial support agent.

At the core of the dual role problem was the ethical tension that staff experienced between the values of human dignity and the values of improving health care through scientific research (Donovan 1981). Often, staff perceived patients on study as vulnerable, dependent, and severely compromised in their ability to accept or refuse what the research protocol indicated (Pellegrino 1981). Workers sought to protect patients whose abilities to reason, judge, and determine their own destinies were markedly reduced (Donovan 1981). To single-mindedly pursue the research protocol was perceived as an infringement upon the humanity of others, reducing the patients to objects of manipulation. The professional staff also felt that the testing protocol interfered with what they considered a more important responsibility, the supportive counseling of patients and family. Humanistic concerns for assisting patients and families in stress and crisis won out over adherence to the prescribed testing protocol.

In a report to the National Cancer Institute, the results of the initial psychosocial testing were acknowledged and a revised protocol was submitted (Vinciguerra et al. 1982). A significant and welcome change for social work staff called for the hiring of professional research assistants to perform the majority of testing and data collection. The focus of the testing itself was to be utilized wherever possible to reduce the extent of patient-completed testing. Finally, the knowledge and expertise of project social work staff was to be captured on the McKegney-Taylor Handicapped Rating Scale, which allows the worker to descriptively rate the individual patient's level of impairment.

In general, staff learned to deal with issues as they arose in their efforts to provide both psychosocial support for patients and psychosocial research with patients. But the fundamental corollary to the research is the enormity and depth of ethical pressures on both the primary researcher and all associated staff (Durant 1981). While the social workers were seeking the value of the individual patient, at times they perceived science as a tool for reducing the importance of the individual. Yet their experience did not deny the potential they saw for science and technology to provide an understanding of what might be done to improve the patients' quality of life (Cullen 1981).

The issues raised through this experience are common to all who attempt medical research. We all need to know (1) that the question asked in a research project is important and (2) that it can be carried out competently with dignity for the patient and with some degree of hope for successful completion (Durant 1981). We must be honest with ourselves about our personal involvement with the study and, moreover, honest with our patients about their expected involvement and contribution (Durant 1981). Concerns for ethics must be inherent in our work and must constitute an area for constant self-examination. As increasingly sophisticated investigations are undertaken and progress emanates from science and technology, the quality of life of patients must remain foremost in our thoughts, and parallel advances in the psychosocial management of cancer must always be present.

REFERENCES

Cullen, J. 1981. "Research Issues in Psychosocial and Behavioral Aspects of Cancer." Paper presented at the American Cancer Society Third National Conference on Human Values and Cancer, April 23-25, Washington, D. C.

Donovan, C. 1981. "The Nurse: Dilemmas with Informed Consent." Paper presented at the American Cancer Society Third National Conference on Human Values and Cancer, April 23-25, Washington, D. C.

Durant, J. 1981. "Dilemmas in Clinical Research: Requiem for a General Resolution." Paper presented at the American Cancer Society Third National Conference on Human Values and Cancer, April 23-25, Washington, D. C.

Pellegrino, E. 1981. "The Moral Foundations for Valid Consent." Paper presented at the American Cancer Society Third National

Conference on Human Values and Cancer, April 23-25, Washington, D. C.

Vinciguerra, V., D. Budman et al. 1984. "Improved Cancer Care through a Home Care Program." Grant #CA-27683-02, Final Summary.

_____. 1982. "Improved Cancer Care through a Home Program." Grant #CA-27683-02.

_____. 1980. "Improved Cancer Care through a Home Program." Grant #CA-27683-01.

22

Diethylstilbestrol: The Psychological Impact of Infertility, Miscarriage, and Stillbirth

Nechama Liss-Levinson

During the three decades spanning 1940 to 1970, at least three million women in the United States were exposed to the drug diethylstilbestrol, also known as DES. This drug was mainly used as a prophylactic agent during pregnancy to prevent miscarriage in women with a previous history of miscarriage or staining.

By 1972 evidence had surfaced relating the mother's ingestion of DES with the development of a rare form of adenocarcinoma in the vagina and/or uterus in a small number of daughters exposed to DES in utero (Herbst et al. 1971). Further investigation revealed that at least 90 percent of the exposed girls had extensive adenosis in the vagina, and a smaller number had numerous irregularities of the cervix and uterus. Extensive screening programs were developed to examine girls and women exposed to DES, and protocols for the appropriate examination of these individuals (including colposcopy, palpation, and multiple smears of both vagina and cervix) were developed (Anderson et al. 1979).

As the generation of women exposed to DES in utero has approached their childbearing years, more attention has been focused on some of the reproductive implications of their DES exposure. Numerous studies have been published recently that indicate high rates of spontaneous abortions, ectopic pregnancies, stillbirths, and premature live births (Barnes et al. 1980; Herbst et al. 1980; Schmidt et al. 1980). Approximately 80 to 85 percent of the DES-exposed women did eventually give birth to full-term healthy infants, as compared with 90 to 95 percent of their nonexposed counterparts. The results relating DES exposure to infertility are equivocal, although DES-exposed daughters report more menstrual difficulties, including anovulation and oligomenorrhea.

As the medical profession considers the physical difficulties faced by these women, it would do well to examine the psychological

impact as well. Obstetricians have often chosen their field because
it is a happy one in which new life is brought into this world. It is a
disappointment to the physician and other medical personnel, as well
as to the expectant family, when the pregnancy ends in fetal wastage.

The medical team must be alerted to the feelings of the parents,
including anger, rage, fear, sadness, and grief. There may be a
special anger here, since the parents may feel that they can attribute
their tragedy to the mother's exposure to DES and, indirectly, to the
medical profession. Their anger may therefore be directed toward
various medical personnel, including the woman's own obstetrician
as a representative of the group. As will be discussed later in this
chapter, the overwhelming angst of the potential grandmother, the
DES mother herself, is another factor to be carefully considered and
dealt with, as appropriate.

For the past three years I have served as a psychological consultant to the Long Island Jewish-Hillside Medical Center DES Screening Program. Working with a nurse-clinician, I have facilitated a
series of rap groups and occasional individual counseling sessions for
women and couples dealing with the impact of DES on their reproductive life. The remainder of this chapter offers (1) specific insights
regarding the psychological impact of DES in dealing with infertility,
miscarriage, and stillbirths and (2) suggestions for the implementation of certain procedures by hospital staff and individual physicians.

INFERTILITY

The greater and greater success of contraception in our society
has bred a generation that expects conception once contraception is
removed. When this does not happen, many assumptions about oneself are challenged. One's own identity, particularly one's sexual
identity, may seem to be at stake. Although one may know all of the
facts regarding the causes of infertility, one may still believe that
only through a successful pregnancy can womanhood or adulthood be
proved.

The pressures may be increased by unwelcome comments by
others, well-meaning and otherwise. In addition, the couple may experience tension over "whose fault is this anyway?" The potential
grandmother, who may have thought that she had resolved her feelings
regarding the DES issue years ago, may now be flooded anew with emotions. Many DES mothers have expressed the feeling that they will
only be vindicated of all guilt once their daughters are able to produce
healthy progeny. The pressures on the young couple and the older
woman are tremendous.

Another difficult issue for the DES couple involves the nature
of some of the treatments suggested to cure the infertility problem.

The physician who suggests various medications and/or hormones must be sensitive to the reaction of the young couple that the specter of DES is being summoned. It does not matter that the drug suggested now is not medically related to DES. For the couple, the dilemma is very real, almost a primal reenactment of one of the major traumatic incidents of their very lives. It is important for the physician in this situation to realize that the couple needs to evaluate their own situation and that there does not have to be one right answer for every individual.

In the past the silence and secrecy surrounding infertility compounded the problems it presented. This silence is being replaced by both knowledge and public discussion of the problem. The physician would do well to be aware of various support groups in this area, such as RESOLVE, which can be used as possible referrals for the couple experiencing infertility problems.

MISCARRIAGE AND STILLBIRTH

A disproportionately high number of DES daughters have miscarriages or stillbirths. One study reported that 40 to 50 percent of first pregnancies for DES-exposed women have unfavorable outcomes (Schmidt et al. 1980). This difficult situation is often worsened by the reluctance of anyone—professional staff or personal friends—to give validity to the event. A miscarriage is often dismissed as unimportant because the woman was not pregnant for very long. A stillbirth is often frightening to others, and everyone would prefer the entire event to disappear without leaving a trace. The parents, on the other hand, have to confront the reality of the tragic event and have a need to mourn their real loss. Those who advise the couple that "it was for the best," that "something was probably wrong with the fetus," or that they can "try again" are missing the essential reality of the situation. The couple mourns not only their physical loss but the loss of all their dreams for that child.

The obstetrician treating a DES-exposed woman can initially inform her of her higher risk category regarding miscarriage, let her know some of the warning signs, and tell her what she might do if such an event seems to be under way. In addition, following a miscarriage or stillbirth medical professionals can give the couple some idea of what to expect in terms of the intensity and range of their feelings and can reassure them that these reactions are normal and acceptable.

Some hospitals have begun to train their staff for dealing with this type of loss and have instituted policies that facilitate the mourning process. The policies may include encouraging the parents to see or touch the stillborn, name the baby, have a burial or service for the baby, and talk about the events with family and friends. It is also important to pay attention to the rooming situation of the patient. Although some experts in this area leave the choice of room arrangements (in the maternity ward or on another floor) up to the woman, I would suggest that the medical team encourage the woman to leave maternity. Many women, when given a choice, may feel that they should be strong and get used to seeing babies, not allowing themselves the permission to experience intensive mourning without immediately dealing with society at large.

For any woman who miscarries or gives birth to a stillborn, there are questions she may ask herself, some of which are unrelated to the physical reality of the event. "What did I do wrong that caused this to happen?" "Should I have taken it easy more often?" "Did I jog too much?" "Was I wrong to lift up my four-year-old daughter?" The medical team must provide the woman and her husband with the facts of the situation in order to alleviate unnecessary guilt and self-recriminations. Information must be presented clearly, concisely, and most important, a number of times. The woman may not initially integrate all that her medical team is telling her.

For the DES family, the guilt that is commonly felt may be intensified and multigenerational. The potential grandmother may blame herself for her daughter's misfortune. The daughter, who has a need to mourn, may feel that she must hide her feelings from her mother at a time when she may need her mother's support. These issues are difficult to resolve, but the medical team should be aware of their interplay and can help to bring them into the awareness of the DES family.

CONCLUSION

The health care team has much to contribute to the woman who is experiencing the traumatic effects of DES exposure in relation to her childbearing capacity. The role of the professional can include (1) providing realistic expectations for the couple regarding the pregnancy; (2) providing accurate information to the couple regarding the miscarriage or stillbirth, thereby clearing up confusion and alleviating useless guilt; (3) providing realistic expectations for the couple regarding both the physical and psychological aftermath of miscarriage or stillbirth; (4) reassuring the couple—and particularly the woman—that the feelings she is experiencing are normal and real and that she is not crazy; (5) providing counseling referrals for individuals or couples who need assistance in resolving their feelings or who are showing pathological reactions; and (6) supporting and encouraging change in hospital procedures aimed at facilitating the grieving process for the couple.

REFERENCES

Anderson, B., et al. 1979. "Development of DES-Associated Clear Cell Carcinoma: The Importance of Regular Screening." Obstetrics and Gynecology 33(3):293-99.

Barnes, A., et al. 1980. "Fertility and Outcome of Pregnancy in Women Exposed to DES in Utero." New England Journal of Medicine 302(11):609-11.

Herbst, A., et al. 1980. "A Comparison of Pregnancy Experience in DES-Exposed and DES-Unexposed Daughters." Journal of Reproductive Medicine 24(2):62-69.

_____. 1971. "Adenocarcinoma of the Vagina: Association of Maternal Stilbestrol Therapy with Tumor Appearance in Young Women." New England Journal of Medicine 284:878-81.

Schmidt, G., et al. 1980. "Reproductive History of Women Exposed to Diethylstilbestrol in Utero." Fertility and Sterility 33:21-24.

BIBLIOGRAPHY

Berezin, N. 1982. After a Loss in Pregnancy. New York: Simon & Schuster.

Borg, S., and J. Lasker. 1981. When Pregnancy Fails. Boston: Beacon Press.

23

Social Service Intervention for the Gynecologic Cancer Patient

Susan Hunsdon

Gynecologic cancer imposes on the patient a regimen of long-term chemotherapy mandated for the treatment of metastic disease and an uncertain, if not negative, prognosis. Five major social service tasks on behalf of this patient population can be defined: (1) helping the patient to vent her initial emotional reactions to her diagnosis; (2) helping her to mobilize her coping strengths to begin chemotherapy; (3) assisting her problem solving, such as planning for the side effects of treatment or successfully interacting with friends and family; (4) helping her to maintain a functional life-style and positive attitude during the course of treatment; and (5) facilitating understanding, communication, and unity of purpose among the patient, family members, and hospital staff during the terminal period of illness. Clearly, these social service tasks must mesh with the team approach to patient care.

The patient care team of the gynecology tumor service at Mount Sinai Hospital in New York City includes physician, oncology nurse, social worker, and clinic administrator. These individuals function as a coordinated unit to facilitate medical treatment. Communication is maintained between staff members, and there is an opportunity during medical rounds for everyone to give input into patient care plans. On the oncology service, there is some blending of roles between physician, nurse, and social worker. The author of this chapper (a social worker) does considerable medical education to prepare the patient for chemotherapy. The doctor and nurse, in turn, address patients' anxieties about treatment and fears of dying. Facts must be sensitively repeated by staff members at a pace that the patient is emotionally able to tolerate. People do not absorb fearful, unpleasant statements at first hearing. There is often initial denial of the physician's explanations. The team works closely with the liaison psychiatry program, which provides consulting psychiatrists for patients who are severely anxious or depressed and which advises staff on the appropriate handling of such patients. The team also cooperates with the hospital home care department in order to plan comprehensive home services for cancer patients.

As the social worker to the gynecology oncology service, I visit a postsurgical patient within a few days after the physician has informed her that she has cancer and will need chemotherapy treatment. When I first enter the patient's hospital room, she may not understand why I am there or what services I might offer. She may never have needed social services in the past. Then, suddenly and inexplicably, she is confronted with a life-threatening illness. During that first visit with me, several emotions may be expressed. Common reactions are tears, anger, denial of the illness, or paralyzing shock. These emotions must be vented before a patient can mobilize her strength for the treatment ahead. It is sometimes easier to share intense feelings with a neutral staff member than to burden relatives who are also in a state of shock and grief. The first stage of working through feelings may last a few days or a few weeks, with a frequent theme being "Why me? What did I do to bring on my cancer?" Women of all ages with gynecologic cancer may turn inward for explanations of their disease, alluding to long-suppressed areas of guilt such as abortions or sexual liaisons. They perceive the cancer as a punishment for such transgressions. Even if it engenders self-blame, finding a meaning for an illness is comforting. It is difficult to accept the notion that cancer strikes in a purposeless, irrational fashion, with no readily identifiable culprit such as a virus or bacterium or life-style. My task as a social worker is to gently buttress physicians' statements that the patient did not cause her illness, that medical science does not know why she has cancer. Although we are not able to satisfy a patient's emotional need for a cause, we can move on and offer hope for treatment.

The second social service task is to help the patient mobilize her coping strengths to begin chemotherapy. Again, the patient may show a range of emotional reactions. There may be resistance and anger to being told that she must accept treatment. This can reactivate childhood conflicts over autonomy and control over one's body. Teenagers are frequently noncompliant patients, because their need to assert independence from authority figures clashes with seemingly arbitrary treatment procedures. Since the chemotherapy physician plays such a crucial role in a patient's life, he or she may arouse primitive emotions and regressive behavior. Some patients view the doctor as a harsh, withholding parent; other patients perceive their physician as a kind, all-powerful figure. It is helpful for the social worker to have gained some knowledge of major developmental events in the patient's life in order to understand her current emotional reactions. A patient may be helped to reflect on the dynamics of her behavior and may be encouraged to eliminate irrational responses that might interfere with her use of treatment. An awareness of a patient's personality patterns enables the social worker to assist staff to meet the patient's needs.

A 34-year-old woman who had led a fairly independent adulthood was treated on our service. Her cancer, however, brought back all the terror of a childhood crisis when her mother abandoned the family. Although patient and mother had been reunited for many years, her renewed fear of being alone led to excessive demands for the presence of the mother or substitute staff members in her hospital room. Once the staff understood the reasons for the patient's behavior, they were able to respond to her emotional needs without anger or misunderstanding.

Some patients react to the need for chemotherapy by assuming as much control as possible over the situation. The social worker can encourage positive efforts such as attention to diet and exercise. When feasible, treatments are scheduled so that patients may continue working or going to school. Maintaining life activities and goals contributes to the sense of control over one's destiny.

Sometimes a patient's response to her diagnosis precipitates a serious depressive reaction, which precludes an effective response to chemotherapy. The social worker and other staff must be alert to this problem and refer the patient for psychiatric help. The psychiatrist may prescribe antidepressants and adjust pain medication for effective emotional stabilization of the patient. Ongoing psychiatric therapy may be needed for patients who are particularly vulnerable to stress.

A third social service task is to assist the patient with problem solving during treatment. The social worker helps the physician and oncology nurse in preparing a patient for the distressing side effects of chemotherapy: hair loss, nausea, and general fatigue. For a woman who has recently undergone a hysterectomy as part of her treatment, chemotherapy is an additional assault on her femininity. How well a patient accepts and adjusts to these bodily changes depends on her self-image and the reactions of those closest to her. It has been my experience that women expect more rejection from husbands and boyfriends then actually occurs. In our society, hair is associated with a woman's feelings of attractiveness and sexual desirability. Patients tell me that after they lose their hair, they cannot bear to look at themselves in the mirror. When I ask how their husbands are feeling, patients often state that their spouse does not care about the hair loss. He is just thankful to have his wife home with him. In fact, there is no need for a woman to look unattractive during chemotherapy. The social worker and nurse may encourage the use of wigs, appro-

priate makeup, and pretty scarves and jewelry. With attention to
rest and nutrition, a woman can look the picture of health during treatment.

Occasionally, a peripheral side effect such as hair loss can be
the catalyst for a depressive reaction. The primary vanity of a 68-
year-old woman was her lovely long hair, which had not been cut for
30 years. She has suffered acute, sustained grief at losing her hair.
This devastating blow to her self-image has not responded to staff or
psychiatric intervention. Sometimes referral to a therapy group is
the most effective strategy for such patients. Groups enable patients
to develop supportive relationships and to share information and ways
of coping with problems. The social worker is also responsible for
making other referrals, as needed, to appropriate agencies for visiting nurse, homemaker services, financial aid, transportation, counseling, and so forth.

Sharing their diagnosis arouses negative feelings among many
women. Some, fearing discrimination, rejection, or pity, prefer not
to inform employers or casual friends of their cancer. The social
worker can help the patient to think through her feelings, separating
irrational fears from realistic assessments. An individual's personality dynamics and typical patterns of interacting with others are key
variables. A 42-year-old divorcee had a history of unsatisfactory
relationships with significant men in her life. Her father was abusive
and her husband an alcoholic. She had developed a pattern of rejecting prospective suitors before they had an opportunity to disappoint
her. Recently, she met a man who appears to have attributes of sensitivity and loyalty, which were missing from her earlier relationships.
This has created a crisis for her, since she fears that if she tells her
new boyfriend that she is undergoing chemotherapy treatment for cancer, he will desert her. Her tendency is to reject him before he can
hurt her. In therapy, we have explored the reasons for her behavior
and have focused on developing new communication patterns in order
to foster a relationship of trust with her new friend.

A serious illness can be the motivating factor that impels a
patient to initiate positive changes in her life. My patients have revealed that they develop new priorities and values when undergoing
treatment. There is a deepening appreciation of family and friends
and an intense awareness of the beauty in one's daily life.

The fourth social service task is to enable the patient to maintain a positive attitude and functional life-style during long-term
treatment. Cancer can be considered a chronic illness, with periodic
critical flareups. The social worker must assess when independent
functioning can be encouraged and when more intensive help is needed.
A crucial aim is to maintain a patient's self-confidence and decision-
making skills. The primary emotional problem during long-term treat-

ment is the danger of losing a sense of purpose in life and hope for the future. Patients complain that they feel like prisoners of the medical setting with constant appointments and blood tests, and they are unable to motivate themselves to continue work, school, or family responsibilities.

A 38-year-old depressed woman has been under chemotherapy treatment for three years. She has gradually forsworn her role as mother and homemaker because of long periods of not feeling well and a sense that her treatment will never end. Her husband has assumed shopping, cleaning, cooking, and child-care responsibilities. Rather than proving helpful, this has left the patient feeling more depressed and lethargic because she has no focus to her day. She fears that her family no longer needs her. With my encouragement, she has begun to regain some of her status within the family. Modest daily goals have been established, such as ironing or cooking one meal in order to foster a sense of accomplishment. When a patient is able to continue her role at home or at work, she feels a sense of control over her life that helps her to more effectively fight her illness.

Once, as an inexperienced social worker, I tried hard to convince a woman to accept a homemaker. Although the patient was very ill and weak, she continued to refuse my offer. Only later did I realize that my efforts were nontherapeutic. By removing her prerogatives within the home, I was robbing this particular woman of her identity and her motivation to battle her illness.

The final social service task is to facilitate understanding, communication, and unity of purpose between the patient, her family members, and hospital staff during the terminal period of her illness. There comes a point during treatment when physician and staff become aware that the patient is not going to get well and that she is entering a terminal stage. This phase may last for several months or up to a year. The content, quality, and consistency of staff communications with the terminally ill patient are significant variables in her tolerance of this final phase. The key to effective interactions with the patient is careful attention to both verbal and nonverbal cues that will guide the staff to the kind of information that she can tolerate concerning her worsening condition. Cassell (1979) has stressed that information given a patient can be considered a "therapeutic tool" for reducing patient uncertainty and providing a basis for action.

The team approach to patient care, while important in earlier treatment phases, becomes crucial during the final stage. There must be communication between team members and mutual respect for each professional's expertise in order to convey to the patient a sense of unity and cohesive planning. This is imperative because patients' verbalizations to staff are frequently contradictory or inconsistent. For example, in an effort to downplay new symptoms, a patient may not mention a new pain or discomfort to her physician for fear of engendering further tests or medical procedures. However, she feels no threat when discussing this symptom with the nurse or social worker. The team may discuss these varying reports and arrive at a consensus concerning their medical and emotional significance.

It has been my observation that patients are seldom able to confront the inevitability of their own death, even in the face of rapidly worsening symptoms. The acceptance noted by Kubler-Ross (1969, 1975, 1981) has not been evident in our patients, especially not in the younger women. The problem of replicating Kubler-Ross's observations lies in her inconsistent use of the term denial. She never precisely defined what she meant by this concept when she described the movement of terminal patients from denial through anger, bargaining, and depression to final acceptance (1969). In a broad discussion of the meaning of denial, Weisman emphasized its multifaceted nature:

> "Denial" now covers almost any situation, act, or verbal expression in which anyone seeks to "avoid reality," or to escape confrontation with something unpleasant and alarming, at least in the opinion of the observer. [1972, p. 58]

Whether or not a person is viewed as denying her illness depends on the mental set of the beholder and the nature of the communication between therapist and patient. The responses of the patient are also conditioned by ethnic and cultural background. Weisman classified denial into three orders as it relates to terminality and the threat of death:

> First-order denial is based upon how a patient perceives the primary facts of illness. Second-order denial refers to the inferences that a patient draws, or fails to draw, about the extension and implications of his illness. Third-order denial is concerned with the image of death itself: denial of extinction. [1972, p. 67]

Although patients may not have manifested first- or second-order denial at earlier stages of treatment, I believe that third-order denial becomes a primary defense mechanism during the terminal phase. It may also be akin to Kubler-Ross's conceptualization of hope, which she states is retained by even the most accepting and realistic patients. Hope gives the terminally ill person a "rationalization" for his suffering and remains a "form of temporary but needed denial" (1969, p. 139).

Denial of impending death may alternate with brief moments of panic and intense grief when the reality of a patient's condition registers emotionally. During these moments of anticipatory grief, the patient derives support and comfort from staff members who are consistent in their responses. The patient may test the concern and expertise of her medical team by asking the same questions repeatedly to different staff members. The terminology and phrasing of staff communications are significant in helping the patient to maintain an attitude of hope and lessening fears of abandonment. For example, the statement, "Your tumor has spread and you appear to have failed this treatment" may convey the same medical information as "There are a few nodules on your liver but we are hoping that further courses of treatment will help." However, for the patient there is a vast difference in the emotional meanings of the two statements. The former conveys staff frustration and almost blames the patient for her treatment failure; the latter reassures the patient that the staff are still actively engaged in helping her fight her illness.

A 52-year-old college professor with terminal ovarian cancer exhibited two defense mechanisms during the early stages of illness: anger and intellectualizing. Her anger was directed at perceived lapses in hospital and staff services. Her intellectual efforts were focused on repeated demands that her physicians share all details of her condition and treatment with her. Her terminal stage is marked by a significant change in her emotional responses. She is now in acute anticipatory grief, with constant tears that overwhelm and perplex her. Rather than focus on her cancer per se, she discusses alleviation of symptoms. She voices certainty that if her vaginal bleeding could be controlled, she would feel stronger and be able to resume her teaching responsibilities. The patient's emotional changes have necessitated sensitive alterations in staff interaction with her. In response to the patient's signals, she is told of efforts to arrest her bleeding. Her rapidly advancing tumor is no longer discussed in detail with her.

In offering services to terminal patients, social workers exercise traditional assessment and communication skills. They are able to clarify the patient's emotional reactions and her primary defenses and to foster effective communication between the patient and her medical team.

Although this chapter focuses on services to patients, families are offered concomitant assistance, particularly when the patient reaches a terminal stage. Two common aspects of intervention with families during this final period involve work with husbands and with teenage children. As the patient's condition worsens, a husband may need assistance to combat his sense of helplessness. His traditional role as protector of his spouse is eroded by an illness that he is unable to control. Indeed, the physician assumes the role of savior. Men may compensate with angry, ineffectual efforts to obtain services or privileges for their wives. They need help to channel their efforts more effectively and assurances that their love and emotional support are powerful forces in their spouses' battles against the disease. A husband may feel occasional anger at his ill wife for increasing his emotional and financial burdens. These angry feelings engender guilt and are repressed, causing unresolved tension. A therapeutic support group is helpful for spouses; they can then share their feelings with others undergoing the same experiences and derive comfort from the knowledge that their anger and resentments are common, acceptable reactions.

Special services are also offered to teenage daughters of patients. Adolescents are typically in the process of establishing their sexual identity and developing a self-image of future wife and mother. When a mother grows ill with gynecologic cancer, a daughter feels particularly vulnerable, since this is the area on which her own current developmental conflict is focused. If a daughter has been unruly or rebellious in the home, she suffers guilt at causing her mother additional problems. Some teenagers overcompensate by assuming their mother's role within the family and taking on responsibilities that interfere with school and rest. When a patient dies, the daughter's emotional conflicts may become acute and may require referral for long-term therapy. The heart of the problem is generally the daughter's confused feelings about her own developing sexuality. The sexual organs, that element of womanhood perceived as positive and life giving, have become the vehicle for her mother's untimely death.

Teenage sons may also endure great stress, particularly if there is no adult male in the home. The ill patient may lean on her son emotionally, expecting him to be husband and father to her. The adolescent boy is then torn between his own desires for mothering and support and the expectation that he be a strong man. When visiting his mother in the hospital, the boy may be frightened by medical procedures that cause his mother pain or discomfort. These may reactivate oedipal conflicts in him at a time when he is sensitive to his own physical development.

In helping teenagers, the social worker must be alert to their identity conflicts and how the stress of an ill mother can aggravate these problems. The adolescent needs encouragement to verbalize fears and feelings, and sufficient home supports must be offered to prevent the children from being overburdened with mother's care.

Staff communication patterns with family members can constitute an important factor in facilitating appropriate familial responses during the final phase of illness. An assessment must be made of relatives' tolerance for grim medical news. Sometimes family members are no better able than the patient to accept full disclosure of prognosis. Indeed, this may foment secrets between the patient and her family at a time when clear, open sharing of feelings must be encouraged. Ideally, patient and family should arrive together at an emotional understanding of her condition. Too often, relatives repress their feelings in a misguided effort to spare anxiety and grief in loved ones. The social worker can facilitate communication between family members through gentle encouragement and demonstration that open discussion causes comfort rather than pain. In addition, a patient's fears of the unknown and of dying may be aggravated if she senses that medical information or decision making is being shared with family members behind her back. This erodes her attempts to maintain an autonomous sense of self, difficult at best for a terminal patient in the medical setting. There are, of course, instances when relatives who function in a guardianship capacity with the young, very elderly, or emotionally disturbed patient should receive more information than the patient herself. The social worker must be actively involved in aiding these family members to plan appropriately for the patient.

A final social work task is to ensure that patient, family, and staff are working toward the same goals. Although these goals become time limited and modest in the terminal stage, unity of purpose can facilitate comfort and peace of mind for the patient. For example, the gynecology oncology service was treating a terminal 62-year-old patient with metastatic endometrial cancer. She had numerous complications, including pleural effusion, leg edema, and diarrhea. The staff assumed that she might wish to be home for a while and enthusiastically initiated complex home care arrangements, including visiting nurse service, oxygen equipment, and provisions for home hyperalimentation. However, in discussion with the patient and her husband, the social worker learned that they were both terrified of the sophisticated equipment. Each further hinted at the fear that the patient might die at home. The husband had been reluctant to share his feelings with his wife in the belief that she would view his not wanting her home as a rejection. However, the wife verbalized similar fears over management of her pain and medical complications at home. The staff was then able to respond to the couple's needs and the patient remained in the hospital, where she died one week later.

The task of providing medical information in a manner that the terminal patient is emotionally able to tolerate requires sensitivity and consistency on the part of the oncology team members. At the same time, staff must avoid distortion of fact and the arousal of unrealistic expectations in patients and family members. Perhaps these communication skills come most readily to the social worker, since a primary professional adage learned early in training is to "begin where the patient is."

In summary, cancer engenders a series of personal losses and challenges: of plans interrupted, relationships threatened, and daily activities attenuated. The social worker must be skilled in recognizing the emotional stresses common among patients during different phases of their diagnosis and treatment. By alleviating psychosocial problems, the social worker can help the patient to fight her illness, tolerate treatments, and—perhaps—reexamine personal priorities. The social worker is an integral member of the oncology team, facilitating communication between patient, family, and medical staff; serving as a link to resources; and addressing the emotional needs of the patient in order to augment successful treatment. If a patient becomes terminal, her comfort is abetted by staff interventions that convey team unity of purpose and assurance that she will not be abandoned emotionally. Staff expertise is required to assess a patient's unique defense patterns rather than impose preconceived notions of what the terminal patient should be feeling or thinking. Although active medical treatment wanes, supportive and therapeutic contacts remain critical factors in alleviating a patient's fear and despair as she faces her own extinction. Communication skills, which play such a vital role in all human activities, are paramount in easing a patient's final separation from consciousness of self and awareness of others.

REFERENCES

Cassell, E. J. 1979. "Telling the Truth to the Dying Patient." In Cancer, Stress, and Death, edited by J. Tache et al., pp. 121–28. New York: Plenum.

Kubler-Ross, E. 1981. Living with Death. New York: Macmillan.

_____. 1975. Death: The Final Stage of Growth. Englewood Cliffs, N.J.: Prentice-Hall.

_____. 1969. On Death and Dying. New York: Macmillan.

Weisman, A. D. 1972. On Dying and Denying. New York: Behavioral.

24

From a Physical to a
Metaphysical Reality

Egilde Seravalli

A few months ago, a dear friend's struggle ended after deep
personal suffering. She was 40 years old.

The ordeal had begun ten years earlier when a breast nodule
was diagnosed as mammary carcinoma. The mastectomy, the radiation therapy, the chemotherapy, and her strong hope for life did not
succeed in dissipating the fear of death. Until the end, she and her
husband's hopes and fears fluctuated every time another surgical procedure had to be performed. The slow but constant growth of the
tumor and the unpredictable recurrences strained their relationship
to the point where a physical and spiritual distance grew between them.
She became more demanding, and he became more tired and self-
defensive.

The first surgery, the removal of one breast, did not seem to
affect their relationship. It was too strong and deep to be altered by
physical impairment. Both of them, however, knew that something
was changing and that their lives would not remain the same. They
realized that their relationship needed to be reorganized as a result
of hidden but conscious anxieties that could not be ignored.

With effort from both sides a new equilibrium was reached, and
their life resumed its natural cycle—but only for a brief time.

Then, another deceitful and malicious nodule appeared in the
other breast. Again, fears, uncertainties, inhibitions, and hopes
brought other subtle changes in their relationship.

Was it really the fear of feeling different—sort of a lesser kind
of woman—that made their life different from what it had been until
that moment? Were the subtle yet dramatic changes the result only
of the removal of her breasts?

Those who find themselves confronting a disease that dashes
their hope for a long life feel naked, suddenly alone with no psycho-

logical defenses to keep them as integral parts of society. The consequences of this new reality could be alleviated if society were willing to overcome the instinctive fear of, and sometimes the inner resistance to, dying.

Eric Cassell has written the following:

> A young woman (with metastatic disease of the breast) had severe pain, and other physical symptoms that caused her suffering. But she also suffered from some threats that were social and from others that were personal and private. She suffered from the effects of the disease and its treatment on her appearance and abilities. She also suffered unremittingly from the perception of the future. . . .
>
> She felt isolated because she was no longer like other people and could not do what other people did. She feared that her friends would stop visiting her. She was sure that she would die. . . .
>
> No person exists without others; there is no consciousness without a consciousness of others, no speaker without hearer, and no act, object, or thought that does not somehow compass others. All behavior is or will be involved with others, even if only in memory or reverie. . . . Furthermore, the extent and nature of a sick person's relationships influence the degree of suffering from a disease. [1982, p. 639]

The one argument that is most difficult to accept is the fear of cancer as the symbol of death. Cancer's presence can stay in our spirit and in our mind; it does not end once the tumor has been taken out. Its root remains hidden, unseen, ready to challenge at any moment, any instant, the serenity that has been acquired with tremendous effort.

When a woman faces a series of mutilative surgeries—mastectomy, oophorectomy, hysterectomy—the problem moves from a physical to a metaphysical reality. At this point, the crucial questions erupt in all their strength, in their crude, naked truthfulness: "Will I live or will I die?" "Will you live or will you die?" Since the impact of such awareness is so strong, we reduce it to a more manageable dimension. As difficult and painful as this approach can be, it is still far less difficult and painful than the crucial point of life and death. There can be no denial that the fear of losing physical attraction is—and should not be—of major concern for the continuation of a love relationship. But there is an aspect of the problem that is beyond sex.

The presence of the tumor seems to tell the patient, "Your time is shorter now—be careful." The shock is such that the person is limited to human problems ("Am I still sexually attractive?") until she is ready to conceive of her own death.

The process advances from a particular reality, the physical one, to a universal reality, the problem of life and death.

In their hearts, my friends knew that the malignancies would not stop growing. Intellectually, however, they did not realize what was happening until the surgeon decided to remove the woman's uterus. He found that she was pregnant. When he learned this news, the husband's anger, frustration, and depression surfaced. Despite his effort to demonstrate love for his wife, he became visibly detached from her. He had been able to cope with every problem, but now he could not cope with the loss of his child. Husband and wife had overcome the difficulties of her ordeal together until the tumor took away his son. At this point, the rebellion hidden in him exploded. Recognizing that he would be alone soon, he lost the last thin hope of living with the illusion of his wife's presence.

From that moment on, the awareness of being no more two—he and she—but three—he and she and the tumor—overwhelmed the final period of her life. Although she continued to depend on her husband and he continued to give her support and caring, the inner changes that the last event had brought on were irreconcilable and were perceived by friends, family, and perhaps by them, too. As in Tolstoy's The Death of Ivan Ilych, they were always with "It, face to face with It, alone with It. . . . And nothing could be done with It except to look at It and shudder" (Tolstoy 1960, p. 134). Or, as Simone de Beauvoir has written, "It is useless to try to integrate life and death, and to behave rationally in the presence of something that is not rational: each must manage as well as he can in the tumult of his feelings" (de Beauvoir 1964, pp. 113-14).

REFERENCES

de Beauvoir, S. 1964. A Very Easy Death. Philadelphia: Warner Books.

Cassell, E. 1982. "The Nature of Suffering and the Goal of Medicine." New England Journal of Medicine 306: 639-45.

Tolstoy, L. 1960. The Death of Ivan Ilych. New York: New American Library.

25

The Importance of the Social Environment for Women with Breast Cancer

Elizabeth J. Clark

In 1982 an estimated 37,300 women in the United States died from breast cancer (American Cancer Society 1981). Also in 1982 approximately 112,000 new cases of breast cancer were diagnosed, and it is currently predicted that one out of every eleven women in the United States will develop breast cancer at some time during their lives (American Cancer Society 1981). Not only is breast cancer the most common type of cancer in women, it is also the leading cause of cancer deaths among women.

Because of the overwhelming nature of the mortality and morbidity data relating to breast cancer, other important data tend to be overshadowed, particularly survival data. Early diagnosis and better treatment have extended survival time considerably. Of women with localized breast cancer, 88 percent are expected to be alive in five years. In addition, 50 percent of women with nonlocalized breast cancer have projected five-year survival rates (American Cancer Society 1981). Another usually unknown statistic is that the estimated number of women presently alive who have undergone mastectomies, generally the treatment of choice for breast cancer, is over 600,000 (Axtell et al. 1976).

In view of these survival statistics, the focus of research regarding the effects of breast cancer must be extended. Like the majority of research in psychosocial oncology in general, most of the previous studies about breast cancer have been concerned with the time period of diagnosis and intensive treatment, particularly the psychological effects of a mastectomy, or with the terminal stage of the illness. Also, with few exceptions (most notably Worden and Weisman 1977), theories and data in the literature tend to indicate that women with breast cancer are at high risk for a variety of personal problems ranging from depression, anxiety, and low self-esteem

(Asken 1975; Maguire et al. 1978; Polivy 1977; Witkin 1978) to sexual problems and family maladjustment (Anderson 1974; Fellner 1973; Klein 1971; Woods 1975). Little attention has been paid to understanding what factors help women successfully readjust to life after the diagnosis of breast cancer.

THE ROLE OF THE SOCIAL ENVIRONMENT

Two areas that appear to be particularly important in adaptation to cancer are the social environment and interpersonal relationships. For example, Berkman and Syme (1979) studied the link between social environment and mortality and found that social and community ties are associated with the risk of mortality and with specific causes of death such as heart disease, cerebrovascular disease, circulatory disorders, and cancer. They examined four sources of social relationships including marriage, family and friends, church membership, and group memberships. With few exceptions, patients with each type of social tie had lower mortality rates than persons lacking such connections.

With regard to interpersonal relationships and cancer, Wortman and Dunkel-Schetter (1979) comprehensively reviewed available research and found two significant consistencies. First, cancer patients appear to experience considerable difficulty in their interpersonal relationships as a function of their disease. Second, there is apparently a positive relationship between the quality of a patient's interpersonal relationships and his or her ability to cope with illness.

Weisman and Worden (1976) observed 120 cancer patients for the three- to four-month period directly after diagnosis (which they call the peak vulnerability period) and found that the presence of strong, interpersonal support was viewed as a psychosocial asset that contributed to successful coping. Weisman's later work (1979) substantiated this finding with the development of a vulnerability scale. Of particular importance was that widows, persons with marital problems, and persons who anticipate little or no support from significant others ranked high on the vulnerability scale.

Specific to breast cancer, 20 years ago Quint (1963) intensively followed 21 breast cancer patients through their first postsurgical year. One finding during this study was that these women experienced "conversational isolationism" because few persons, lay or professional, were willing to talk with them regarding the problems relating to breast cancer and/or the possibility of death.

More recently, Jamison, Wellisch, and Pasnau (1978) found that in a sample of 41 mastectomy patients, women who reported better emotional adjustment also perceived their spouses, children, and the health care personnel who cared for them as more supportive than did women with lower self-reported adjustment.

Another study (Bloom, Ross, and Burnell 1978), this one interventional in design, compared two groups of women who had undergone mastectomies. One group (N = 18) received standard medical services and the other group (N = 21) participated in an intervention program that provided social support. The intervention group received information, education about diagnosis and treatment, and counseling. At follow-up, the researchers concluded that the intervention program had a long-term positive effect.

Woods and Earp (1978) studied postmastectomy patients four years after their surgery and found that social supports available to the women had a buffering effect and seemed to influence their quality of life. The effect was apparent whether social supports were defined as someone available for listening or someone who potentially could give help.

In view of the limited data available on the successful readjustment to life after the diagnosis of breast cancer, the study described below was undertaken. It attempts to identify factors that facilitate positive adaptation and documents the importance of the patient's social environment.

DESCRIPTION OF THE STUDY

As part of a larger research study regarding social support and cancer (Clark 1982), 46 women with breast cancer, referred by physicians to a hospital intervention program, were followed for 18 months. Among other components of the program such as education and counseling, medical social workers conducted ongoing psychosocial assessments and recorded relevant data of needs, problem areas, and levels of social support and psychosocial functioning. Demographic, medical, social, and psychological data were gathered and all contacts with the patient and/or family were recorded.

Social support was directly measured via a social network perspective, with the trained medical social workers rating the type and amount of support patients received from significant others (spouse, family, friends, coworkers, clergy, physicians, and other health care professionals). Patients' levels of adaptation were measured by use of a Cancer Adaptation Score, which included adaptation to treatment, to impaired physical functioning, emotional functioning, and maintenance of social and occupational roles.

TABLE 1

Distribution of Sample by Age

Age	Number	Percentage of Sample
Less than 30	2	4.3
30–34	4	8.7
35–44	6	13.1
45–54	9	19.6
55–64	14	30.4
65–74	8	17.4
75 and over	3	6.5

Note: Total number = 46.

CHARACTERISTICS OF THE SAMPLE

The women ranged in age from 27 to 80 years (see Table 1 for distribution by age). Ten women were under 40 years of age and eight women were over age 70.

Twenty-seven of the women were married, 11 were widowed, 5 were divorced, and 3 were single. Of the 46, 17 (37 percent) were housewives and held no other occupational position, and 15 (32.6 percent) were professional or clerical workers. The rest were skilled or unskilled manual workers or machine operators. The women had received various combinations of treatment including surgery, radiation therapy, and chemotherapy or hormonal treatment. However, 39 (85 percent) had undergone at least one mastectomy.

FINDINGS

For the total sample of 46 breast cancer patients, there was a moderate, positive association between level of social support and level of adaptation to cancer ($r = .34$, $p = .01$). When the relationship between support and adaptation is compared with other types of cancer (data from the larger study, Clark 1982), patients with breast cancer and patients with gynecologic cancer (including cancer of the cervix, endometrium, and/or ovary) had the highest level of adaptation (see Table 2). This means that as a group, they adapted better to the illness of cancer than did patients with colon/rectal cancer,

TABLE 2

Comparison of Social Support and Adaptation to Cancer by Site of Cancer

| | Level of Social Support | | | | | | Level of Adaptation | | | | | |
| | Low | | Moderate | | High | | Low | | Moderate | | High | |
Site	Number	Per cent	Number	Per cent	Number	Per cent	Number	Per cent	Number	Per cent	Number	Per cent
Breast (N = 46)	12	26	17	37	17	37	7	15	16	35	23	50
Cervix/endometrium/ovary (N = 12)	2	17	5	42	5	42	2	17	5	42	5	42
Colon/rectum (N = 15)	8	53	0	—	7	47	7	47	4	27	4	27
Hodgkin's/lymphoma (N = 12)	4	33	1	8	7	58	4	33	2	17	6	50
Leukemia (N = 13)	3	23	7	54	3	23	4	31	2	15	7	54
Lung (N = 31)	9	29	10	32	12	39	17	55	11	35	3	10

Note: Raw percentages are used, and table does not sum to 100 percent because of rounding error. Total number = 129.

lung cancer, leukemia, or Hodgkin's disease. Fifty percent of the breast cancer patients were in the high adaptation category and 42 percent of those with gynecologic cancer were in that category. When the percentages for moderate and high categories were combined, the percentages were 85 percent for breast cancer patients and 84 percent for patients with cancer of the cervix, endometrium, and/or ovary.

Previous research has not shown psychosocial distress to be consistently site specific for the cancer population (Weisman and Worden 1976). However, one study (American Cancer Society 1979) found that lung cancer patients reported the most negative impact of the illness on their lives. This is consistent with the current study results, which found only three patients (10 percent) with lung cancer in the high adaptation category. Patients with colorectal cancer also appeared to have a lower level of adaptation.

Some cancers seem to be more easily acceptable to the general public than other cancers. This could be due to several causes. Types of cancer with the possibility of cure or good control (such as early-stage breast and cervical cancers) are fairly acceptable. However, types of cancer that still have generally negative prognoses (such as lung cancer) may cause other persons to adopt a fatalistic and negative attitude, thereby decreasing available emotional support for the patient. Also, types of cancers that result in little change of appearance are more acceptable than those requiring mutilating surgery, such as some of the head and neck cancers. These differences could contribute to the amount of support a patient receives and, subsequently, his or her adaptation to cancer.

AGE AND ADAPTATION TO CANCER

In the larger research study (Clark 1982), the variable of age was significantly linked to the variable of social support. There was a negative relationship indicating that as a person advances in age, his or her social support diminishes. This was especially true for the aged widow. However, when the variable of social support was controlled, the effect of age on adaptation to cancer was positive, indicating that older persons adapt better to cancer than younger persons. This was particularly true for breast cancer patients (see Table 3). None of the women under 35 years of age fell in the high adaptation category. In contrast, none of the three women who were over 75 years of age (and all of whom were widowed) fell in the low adaptation category. The younger women had more difficulty adapting to breast cancer than the older women. The group with the highest level of adaptation, 71.4 percent (N = 10), were women between the

TABLE 3

Comparison of Social Support and Adaptation to Cancer by Age

Age	Level of Social Support						Level of Adaptation					
	Low		Moderate		High		Low		Moderate		High	
	Number	Per-cent	Number	Per-cent	Number	Per-cent	Number	Per-cent	Number	Per-cent	Number	Per-cent
Less than 35	1	16.7	4	66.7	1	16.7	1	16.7	5	83.3	0	—
35–44	1	16.7	1	16.7	4	66.7	1	16.7	2	33.3	3	50.0
45–54	3	33.3	2	22.2	4	44.4	1	11.1	4	44.4	4	44.4
55–64	3	21.4	3	21.4	8	57.1	2	14.3	2	14.3	10	71.4
65–74	2	25.0	6	75.0	0	—	2	25.0	2	25.0	4	50.0
75 and over	2	66.7	1	33.3	0	—	0	—	1	33.3	2	66.7

Note: Raw percentages are used. Total number = 46.

ages of 55 and 64 years. This finding is consistent with that of Jamison, Wellisch, and Pasnau (1978), who found that younger women with breast cancer (under age 45) had more problems than older women (over age 45). The younger women in their study considered a mastectomy as having a more detrimental effect on their sex lives.

Another explanation for this finding might be the fact that cancer in the older person is more common and, in some ways, more acceptable to the patient as well as to other persons. Cancer in the young person is seen as especially tragic, and this attitude could make it more difficult for the young person to adapt to the disease. Older persons also may have fewer family and work-related obligations, which could facilitate the process of adaptation.

Two case examples are representative of these findings.

Case 1

Mrs. D, a very attractive 27-year-old woman, discovered a small lump in her breast. Upon biopsy, it was found to be malignant, and she was admitted to the hospital for preparation for a mastectomy. Mrs. D was married and the mother of two small children. She did not work outside the home. She had been a high school beauty queen and was particularly proud of her appearance. She feared she would lose her husband's affection and others' admiration if she lost a breast. Her husband and family were caring and reassuring, but Mrs. D kept delaying the surgery, vacillating between accepting the operation and refusing it. She became depressed and agitated. Counseling was requested.

It was obvious that Mrs. D's identity was closely aligned to her physical appearance. Also, owing to her young age, nurses and other health care professionals saw Mrs. D's case as especially tragic. This attitude was repeatedly related to Mrs. D in verbal and nonverbal ways. People spoke about how unfair it was that someone so young should have any type of cancer and that someone so attractive should have breast cancer. Nurses close to her age became uneasy when caring for her because the situation was "too close to home" for them. These attitudes compounded the problem for Mrs. D. In addition, her surgeon had become exasperated and felt that valuable time was being lost. The social worker spoke with the physician about the possibility of breast reconstruction. He had not previously mentioned this option to Mrs. D, but he agreed that it was feasible. A consultation with a plastic surgeon was arranged. It was also arranged for Mrs. D to meet with a nurse who had undergone a mastectomy and reconstructive surgery. The nurse was very open and helpful and showed Mrs. D what her reconstructed breast looked like. After this visit, and with the prospect of reconstructive surgery, Mrs. D agreed to the removal of her breast. Several weeks later the reconstructive surgery was performed. However, when adjuvant chemotherapy was recommended later, Mrs. D adamantly refused because she would not risk losing her hair.

Case 2

Mrs. R, a 79-year-old widow of Irish descent, was admitted to the hospital with probable breast cancer. She had been housecleaning and, while turning her mattress, had bumped her breast. This caused severe pain. The pain persisted and she went to her family doctor. During the examination he noted a large lump under her arm, which Mrs. R said she had had for several months. When asked why she had not had it checked, she stated she was afraid it might be cancer. Her diagnostic work-up confirmed the suspicion of regionalized breast cancer. When the surgeon explained the operation (a mastectomy) that he would perform the following day, Mrs. R began to cry and kept repeating, "Not my breast, not my breast." She was tearful and depressed prior to surgery, and this persisted during her postoperative stay. Nurses and other health care professionals expressed surprise at Mrs. R's reaction. They felt that at age 79, losing a breast would not be too important. Mrs. R was embarrassed by her lopsided appearance and was much relieved when a Reach to Recovery volunteer visited and gave her a temporary prosthesis to wear home.

Mrs. R had come to the United States when she was 14 and had married at 16. After having three children, she divorced her first husband, something seldom heard of during that era. She worked in a factory for several years to support her children. At age 38 she remarried. Her second marriage had been a happy one until her husband's death six years earlier. Since then she had lived alone in a three-room apartment in federal housing for the elderly. She was remarkably alert and independent. She was proud of her independence and of her housekeeping abilities. She had friends and a limited social life at her apartment house. Two of her children lived in the area, and she had fairly frequent contact with them.

Upon discharge, Mrs. R was scheduled for six weeks of radiation therapy. Her children decided that Mrs. R could not care for herself any longer (and particularly get to her radiation appointments), so Mrs. R reluctantly went to stay with one of her daughters. However, she refused to give up her own apartment. She withstood the radiation therapy remarkably well and spoke frequently of her goal of returning to her own apartment when treatment was finished. Upon the completion of her radiation therapy, it was decided she should have a cycle of chemotherapy. Mrs. R was cooperative about her treatment, but she was disappointed that she would have to continue living with her daughter for a little longer. Her daughter had grown somewhat resentful of having the responsibility for the total care of her mother. She felt her brother and sister should take a turn in caring for Mrs. R. As they had done for most of their lives, Mrs. R and her daughter clashed on many issues, and the time Mrs. R spent with the daughter was not particularly pleasant. She especially disliked her daughter's bossiness—always telling her what and when she should eat and insisting that she get more rest. Despite these problems, Mrs. R did not manage to return to her apartment for almost eight months. Her children were unhappy that "she was so stubborn" and insisted on living alone. By this time, metastasis was noted in Mrs. R's bones and lungs. All definitive treatment was stopped, and the goal became one of keeping her comfortable. With the help of the Visiting Nurse Association, Mrs. R managed to stay in her own apartment for two months and she was delighted to be home. She was direct in talking about the fact that she was going to die and numerous times stated that she was ready. When her pain became too much to manage at home, she was admitted to the hospital where she died a few days later.

MARRIAGE AND ADAPTATION TO CANCER

Marriage did not provide a protective buffer. Of the 46 women, 27 were married at the time of the study. Despite somewhat higher levels of support, married patients adapted no better than their non-married counterparts: 44 percent of the married women fell in the high adaptation category compared with 58 percent of the nonmarried women. Part of the explanation for this may be the greater family responsibilities of the married population and their concomitant family problems. In addition, 19 percent of the married patients reported problems of marital communication and family discord. This is similar to the findings of a study by Gordon et al. (1977), in which a group of 136 cancer patients was asked to indicate their major problems. The second most frequently reported problem was the absence of open communication within the family. Discussion of emotions between patients and family members is often difficult. The two cases described below illustrate different communication patterns. It is interesting to note the age and marital status differences in the two cases.

Case 3

Mrs. J was a 34-year-old woman, married and the mother of three small children. While nursing her youngest child, she developed a breast infection. Routine treatment proved unsuccessful and when the child was nine months old, a diagnostic work-up was done that disclosed metastasized breast cancer. Radiation therapy was begun, and later Mrs. J had several cycles of chemotherapy.

Mr. J was not able to accept his wife's illness or the seriousness of the disease. He constantly downplayed her condition, refusing to discuss or hear what the physician and other health care professionals were saying. He repeatedly told them they were making too much of his wife's problem. He expected his wife to maintain her prediagnosis level of functioning. In fact, his denial took the form of adding more duties to Mrs. J's role. He wanted her to entertain more and to help more with the business they owned.

Mr. and Mrs. J were not close geographically or emotionally to other family members. Over the years, Mr. J had managed to alienate most of his wife's relatives. When they realized the seriousness of Mrs. J's illness, they wanted to help. They lived several hours away but asked to take the two older children, ages four and eight, for the summer. Mr. J refused, claiming his wife could manage just fine. He also refused to have her relatives come to help.

As Mrs. J's condition worsened, Mr. J's expectations became more and more unreasonable. However, Mrs. J never complained about her husband. If he accompanied her to medical appointments (which was rare), she always reported she was feeling well and had no problems. If she came alone or with a volunteer driver, she was more open about her physical problems but always defended her husband and his beliefs. Finally, Mrs. J could no longer maintain the household and care for the children. Homemaker services were arranged and child care was provided. But Mr. J wanted no evidence of this when he came home. The distance between Mr. and Mrs. J continued to grow, and in the final months of her life her only source of support was the care provided by the health professionals. She died in a hospital. Mr. J was not present. He had never been able to accept her illness or to provide her with support or understanding. In his eyes, Mrs. J had failed him.

Case 4

Miss E was a 69-year-old woman, never married, who had retired seven years earlier from her job as a salesclerk. She had lived with her parents until they died, her father from heart disease and her

mother from a questionable malignancy, when they were in their
eighties. At their death, Miss E moved in with a sister and an older
brother who was a retired priest. Another married sister lived nearby
and they visited often. A younger sister had died previously from
breast cancer. In March Miss E was seen for weight loss, cough,
fatigue, and shortness of breath. A pleural biopsy showed metastatic
adenocarcinoma compatible with a primary tumor of the right breast.
Bone and brain scans were normal at that time. She was begun on a
chemotherapy regimen, which continued until her death 16 months
later.

The family was exceptionally close and openly and realistically
discussed Miss E's illness. They had strong religious beliefs from
which they drew much comfort. Miss E's condition continued to de-
teriorate slowly from the time of her diagnosis, but she was able to
maintain a near-normal level of activity for many months and managed to go on a family vacation in August.

In June her brother celebrated his fiftieth year in the priesthood.
While struggling with back pain from bone metastasis, Miss E was
able to participate in the festivities. She died at home, as the family
wished.

Miss E's family support never waivered. Oftentimes, all three
of Miss E's siblings would accompany her to doctor appointments.
All were interested in her condition, her treatment, and her progress.
Miss E, her brother, and her sisters had openly discussed cancer and
dying and were as well prepared as possible for her death. While they
realized from the time of her diagnosis that Miss E's breast cancer
could not be cured, they wanted her to live as fully as possible in the
time she had remaining, and she did.

OCCUPATION AND ADAPTATION TO CANCER

Higher occupational ranking served a protective function aiding
in adaptation to breast cancer, with women in high statuses (such as
professionals and administrators) receiving more support than women
in lower-level positions (such as factory workers). This was particularly true for housewives. Only 35 percent of the housewives fell in
the high adaptation category, while over 66 percent of the professional
women had high levels of adaptation. Similarly, over 66 percent of
the professional women had high levels of social support, while only
29 percent of the housewives had high support. Several factors might
help to explain these results. First, for reasons such as higher educational levels or better financial resources, professional women
might be more capable of seeking and/or developing needed support
systems or might be better able to utilize what is available. Also,

women in higher statuses might experience higher levels of tolerance toward their illness (that is, changing work schedules, available sick time, and so forth) than women who work in a factory or lower-level job.

SUMMARY

Several social factors—age, marital status, and occupational status—that seem to have an impact on women's adaptation to breast cancer have been discussed. Breast cancer patients as a group appear to adapt better to their illness than do patients with other types of cancer, such as colorectal and lung cancers. Yet, with one out of every 11 women predicted to get breast cancer in their lifetimes, it is important that research be expanded to gain a better understanding of adaptation to this disease.

First, there must be more awareness of the progress that is being made in the treatment of breast cancer. Advances in cancer control have helped transform cancer from an acute to a chronic disease. Along with chronicity has come concern for the quality of the survival time of patients. Particularly salient is the large number of women who have had breast cancer, which is now controlled, and who are learning to live successfully with a chronic illness as life-threatening and as socially stigmatized as cancer. Understanding how these persons adapt to living with this knowledge is crucial for an understanding of the psychosocial problems of chronic disease in general.

This approach is not meant to negate the fact that women with breast cancer have a difficult time during the periods of diagnosis and intensive treatment, particularly with adjustment to the surgical procedure of mastectomy. But as Worden and Weisman noted,

> Overemphasis of sexual implications following breast surgery may lead to underemphasis of more significant psychosocial concerns. . . . Cosmetic problems are real and we do not minimize the damaged body image in anyone. But psychosocial rehabilitation for breast patients does not stop when a prosthesis is fitted. [1977, p. 175]

CLINICAL IMPLICATIONS

The social environment of cancer patients and the quality of their interpersonal relationships are important considerations in the rehabilitation process. Current research indicates that an individual's ability to adapt to cancer can be augmented by members of his or her social network of family, friends, coworkers, and health care professionals.

Several years ago, Cassel pointed out that "it seems more feasible to attempt to improve and strengthen the social supports rather than to reduce the exposure to stressors" (1976, p. 121). We may not yet be able to prevent cancer, but we do have the potential for helping people live successfully with this disease.

Early assessment must include an evaluation of a patient's social environment. Follow-up care should take into account the type and amount of support available from the patient's interpersonal relationships. Patients can be encouraged and helped to mobilize whatever resources are available to them, and those at high risk to poor adaptation owing to little social support should be referred for more intensive professional intervention.

REFERENCES

American Cancer Society. 1981. Cancer Facts and Figures, 1982. New York: American Cancer Society.

_____. 1979. Report on the Social, Economic, and Psychological Needs of Cancer Patients in California. San Francisco: American Cancer Society.

Anderson, R. 1974. "Notes of a Survivor." In The Patient, Death and the Family, edited by S. B. Troub, pp. 73-82. New York: Charles Scribners.

Asken, M. 1975. "Psychoemotional Aspects of Mastectomy: A Review of the Literature." American Journal of Psychiatry 132: 56-59.

Axtell, L. M., et al. 1976. Cancer Patient Survival: Report No. 5, Department of Health, Education and Welfare Publication no. NIH 77-992. Washington, D.C.: U.S. Government Printing Office.

Berkman, L. F., and S. L. Syme. 1979. "Social Networks, Host Resistance and Mortality: A Nine-Year Follow-up Study of Alameda County Residents." American Journal of Epidemiology 109(2): 186-204.

Bloom, J. R., R. D. Ross, and G. Burnell. 1978. "The Effects of Social Support on Patient Adjustment after Breast Surgery." Patient Counseling and Health Education 1:50–59.

Cassel, J. 1976. "The Contribution of the Social Environment to Host Resistance." American Journal of Epidemiology 104(2): 107–22.

Clark, E. J. 1982. "The Role of Social Support in Adaptation to Cancer." Dissertation Abstracts International 42:12.

Fellner, C. H. 1973. "Family Disruption after Cancer Care." American Family Physician 8:169–72.

Gordon, W. I., et al. 1977. "The Psychosocial Problems of Cancer Patients: A Retrospective Study." Paper presented at the American Psychological Association meeting, San Francisco, September 1977.

Jamison, K. R., D. K. Wellisch, and R. O. Pasnau. 1978. "Psychosocial Aspects of Mastectomy: I." American Journal of Psychiatry 135:432–36.

Klein, R. 1971. "A Crisis to Grow On." Cancer 28:1660–65.

Maguire, G. P., et al. 1978. "Psychiatric Problems in the First Year after Mastectomy." British Medical Journal 1:963–65.

Polivy, J. 1977. "Psychological Effects of Mastectomy on a Woman's Feminine Self-Concept." Journal of Nervous and Mental Disorders 164:2.

Quint, J. C. 1963. "The Impact of Mastectomy." American Journal of Nursing 63:88–92.

Weisman, A. D. 1979. Coping with Cancer. New York: McGraw-Hill.

Weisman, A. D., and J. W. Worden. 1976. "The Existential Plight in Cancer: Significance of the First 100 Days." International Journal of Psychiatry in Medicine 7(1):1–15.

Witkin, M. 1978. "Psychosexual Counseling of the Mastectomy Patient." Journal of Sex and Marital Therapy 4:20–28.

Woods, N. F. 1975. "Influences on Sexual Adaptation to Mastectomy.' Journal of Obstetric, Gynecological and Neonatal Nursing 4:33-37.

Woods, N. F., and J. L. Earp. 1978. "Women with Cured Breast Cancer." Nursing Research 27(5):279-85.

Worden, J. W., and A. D. Weisman. 1977. "The Fallacy of Post-mastectomy Depression." American Journal of Medical Science 273:169-75.

Wortman, C., and C. Dunkel-Schetter. 1979. "Interpersonal Relationships and Cancer: A Theoretical Analysis." Journal of Social Issues 35(1):120-55.

26

The Urethral Syndrome: A Threat to Body Image

Selwyn Z. Freed

The female urethra is the one structure that, more than any other, brings urologists and gynecologists together. Paraurethral glands, homologues of the prostate gland in the male, are localized mainly in the dorsolateral portion of the distal third of the urethra and are an integral part of the anterior vaginal wall. Its dysfunction led to the appeal to both disciplines—urology and gynecology—"Come, let us reason together."

A diagnosis of urethral syndrome is the most common one for women presenting in the urologist's office. A significant number of patients have already consulted other urologists and gynecologists, a testimony not only to the syndrome's prevalence but also to the frustration in therapy for both patient and doctor. In one series of 1,500 new patients seen each year (male and female), approximately 500 were women with the urethral syndrome (Roberts and Smith 1968).

Considerable confusion is caused by lumping this syndrome together with true bacterial cystitis. In addition, the evidence indicates that a number of separate—though sometimes overlapping—diseases of the urethra also provoke the syndrome. By definition, then, urethral syndrome should be limited to a condition characterized by such urinary symptoms as frequency, dysuria, urgency (perhaps to the point of incontinence), and a sense of inadequate relief after voiding, along with a rather vague discomfort that may be mainly suprapubic or perineal. The urinary symptoms and physical discomforts may be present singly or together, but a most important criterion is a sterile urine (although this does not necessarily mean that infection plays no role). Dyspareunia is often present. The syndrome may be episodic or almost continuous, may alternate with or begin with true bacterial cystitis, and may occur at all ages. It has been referred to by many other names, including irritable bladder, cystalgia, neuralgia of the bladder, cystospasm, trigonitis, rheumatic urethritis, abacterial cystitis, female prostatitis, Reizblase, and <u>cystalgies à urine claires</u>.

Possible etiologies include (1) urethral obstruction, (2) urethritis (bacterial or nonspecific), (3) purulent periurethral glands, (4) neurogenic dysfunction, (5) senile changes, (6) allergy, (7) psychoneurosis, (8) urethral diverticulum, (9) interstitial cystitis, (10) pseudomembranous trigonitis, (11) bladder neck pseudopolypi, (12) urethral-hymenal fusion, (13) gastrointestinal pathology, (14) congested gemelli muscles, and (15) "hygienic" detergents and enzymes.

Urethral diverticulum and interstitial cystitis are pertinent only in that they can cause similar symptoms. However, careful examination should rule them out. Pseudomembranous trigonitis and bladder neck pseudopolypi are, in the author's opinion, so commonly seen in the absence of any symptoms that they cannot be invoked as etiological factors. They cause no dysfunction. Urethral-hymenal fusion is a pathological entity but may be responsible for bacterial cystitis, not urethral syndrome. Colonic disease, congested gemelli muscles, and excessive use of vaginal detergents have all been reported as causes of the syndrome and can be ruled out by simple history and physical examination; they are of anecdotal interest only. Much more attention should be directed at the first seven suggested etiologies.

Anatomic obstruction in the urethra of these women has been demonstrated by uruflowmetry and <u>bougie à boules</u>. This has been attributed to the formation of fibroelastic tissue in the distal urethrovaginal septum by Richardson (1969) and to collagen formation by Evans (1971). Reduction in elasticity is considered the culpable factor. Bladder neck obstruction, meatal stenosis, or moderate diminution of the normal range of urethral caliber are probably not important.

It would seem logical that colonization of bacteria in the urethra should at least be a factor in this syndrome. One bacteriological study of the urethra in women with sterile urine cultures showed that 100 percent contained bacteria in the first centimeter, which included the meatus. Moving proximally, the bacterial counts diminished until only 54 percent of cases had bacteria in the segment adjacent to the vesical orifice. Diphtheroids predominated, but 27 percent of the urethras contained E. coli and other pathogens. It is probable that nonresistance of the urethral mucosa rather than a lack of available pathogens determines their presence (Cox 1966). Another study found that introital cultures were indicative of urethral bacterial flora, and it was concluded that this could cause the urethral syndrome (O'Grady et al. 1970). Doubt was cast on this hypothesis by Bruce and associates (1974), who found that a significant number of control women had pathogenic bacteria in their introital, vaginal, and urethral cultures. However, it was conceded that a higher incidence of pathogenic bacteria occurred in women with recurrent urethritis. Postmenopausal women, both controls and patients, had the highest incidence of pathogens. However, it was not clear that women with true cystitis were separated, and it continues to be a common experience to find introital and urethral pathogens in women with no symptoms and none in sufferers.

How about other organisms, especially those that are sexually transmitted? Trichomonas vaginalis has been found in the urethra (Kean and Wolinska 1956), while the urethral syndrome has been associated with chlamydial infection (Tait, Rees, and Jameson 1978).

Certainly, the paraurethral glands can become infected and every urologist has, at times, been able to observe the expression of purulent material into the urethral lumen. This has been called a female prostatitis (Moore 1960). There is much doubt, however, that this is a consistent finding in the urethral syndrome.

The epithelium of the distal part of the urethra undergoes a process of maturation under the stimulus of estrogens. These changes are, of course, recognized in the vagina, and just as deficiency of estrogen may result in a "senile" vaginitis, so the same deficiency may lead to a "senile" distal urethritis. Such a urethra is rigid, inelastic, and easily inflamed. Both changes, in the vagina as well as in the urethra, may be reversed by estrogens (Smith 1972). Just as respiratory allergy and inflammation go hand in hand, so urinary tract allergy and inflammation are believed by some to have the same relationship (Eisenstaedt 1951, Horesh 1976).

Functional disturbance of the female urethra (and bladder) must certainly be considered in any study of urethral syndrome. Tanagho and Miller (1973) reported a markedly increased amplitude of the urethral pressure profile seen in female patients with recurrent cystitis and meatal stenosis. But Hojsgaard (1976) found no significant difference between the patients with meatal stenosis and normal controls. This challenged the entire concept of static obstruction as a factor in the urethral syndrome. However, bladder instability (Farrar et al. 1976) and especially external sphincter spasticity (Raz and Smith 1976, Tanagho et al. 1971), would seem to have more merit. Elevated tone of the pelvic muscles provokes compensatory inhibition of the detrusors by its inhibitory action on the parasympathetics. On the other hand, low tone of pelvic muscles and external sphincter results in facilitation of bladder contraction. Thus, any factor that can increase the tonic activity of the external sphincter will produce inhibition of detrusor contractions. In severe cases, it may result in complete retention of urine; in milder cases, merely frequency or slowing of the stream, the beginning of urethral syndrome. Urodynamic assessment of 43 women with the urethral syndrome was carried out by Lipsky (1977). He, too, found an incomplete relaxation or spasm of the external striated sphincter, but this was mostly in younger women. Another type of obstruction was found mainly in postmenopausal women, namely, a narrow distal segment of the urethra. It should be noted, however, that in one-third of the patients neither an organic nor functional disturbance of micturition or detrusor was found.

One cannot treat any significant number of women with urethral syndrome without being impressed by their anxiety, emotional disturbance, and—sometimes—neurotic behavior. This has been widely attributed to their urinary discomfort. But other patients with urinary difficulty do not behave this way, and it is difficult to avoid the strong suspicion that for many it is a part of the syndrome, if not the underlying cause. Association between urinary symptoms and emotional disturbance is commonplace, as everyone knows. The bladder is commonly a target organ for the neurotic patient. There are numerous references to this association in the literature (Hafner, Stanton, and Guy 1977; Rees and Farhoumand 1977; Straub, Ripley, and Wolf 1949). Rees and Farhoumand used three psychometric tests (the Eysenck Personality Questionnaire, the Marked Anxiety Inventory, and the Middlesex Hospital Questionnaire), which revealed significant differences such as marked obsessionality and clinical anxiety in particular between patients and controls. A psychoanalytic study of women with urethral syndrome was conducted by Chertok and colleagues in France (1977). They identified two groups: those who tend to be overly passive, depressed, and resigned to life's misfortunes, and those who tend to be active, domineering, and tyrannical.

Certainly, the myriad suggested etiologies of the urethral syndrome support the conviction that it is no single disease. Of course, this must be borne in mind before considering the various therapies, which include (1) urethral dilatation, (2) internal urethrotomy, (3) urethroplasty (Richardson 1969), (4) external urethrotomy, (5) transurethral resection (TUR) of bladder neck, (6) Y-V plasty, (7) meatotomy, (8) antibiotic (systemic), (9) antiseptic (local), (10) suppository (Furacin), (11) bladder instillation (Argyrol), (12) periurethral gland unroofing, (13) periurethral treatment with steroids, (14) urethral estrogens, (15) antihistamines, (16) fulguration of bladder neck polypi, (17) fulguration of trigone and/or urethra, (18) hymenoplasty, (19) treatment with triamcinolone acetamide, (20) massage of gemelli muscles, (21) psychotherapy, and (22) pharmacological approaches.

All of these therapies have adherents. All claim a cure rate of between 60 percent to 95 percent and an average of approximately 70 percent. Most patients are treated with urethral dilatation. Compulsively chosen by the urological community, this procedure has been likened to a marginally misplaced phallic thrust. Although 60 to 70 percent of women report significant relief from this therapy, it seems to bear little relation to the findings on calibration with bougie à boules. Antibacterials and anticholinergics help a significant number of patients, but local antiseptics appear to be worthless. Internal urethrotomy and Richardson-type urethroplasty are popular and logical choices; cure rates in some hands are high. Meatotomy may help a few, but I mention TUR of bladder neck and Y-V plasty only to reject these procedures, as I have rarely seen obstruction at the bladder neck. Periurethral gland unroofing may help the few women who have purulent exudate from this (Leiter 1973; Reiser 1968), but I condemn fulguration of bladder neck polypi, the trigone, or the urethra itself as worthless and perhaps harmful. Antihistamines may be worth trying in selected patients, and I must admit having had a few patients who seemed to respond. I have had no experience with the submucosal injection of triamcinolone acetamide around Skene's glands (Altman 1976), but administration of estrogens locally in post-menopausal women has been occasionally rewarding.

Psychotherapy? Yes, it helps. But it does not have to be in-depth psychoanalysis. A significant percentage of patients can be reached by reassurance and comforting, kind words from a compassionate urologist or gynecologist.

In summary, the urethral syndrome is probably a number of different diseases. No one therapy (and perhaps none) can be trusted. Efforts to identify the specific etiology for appropriate therapy can be rewarding. There can be no substitute for a good history, physical, cultures, urethroscopy, and urodynamic assessment.

REFERENCES

Altman, B. L. 1976. "Treatment of Urethral Syndrome with Triamcinolone Acetamide." Journal of Urology 116:583.

Bruce, A. W., P. Chadwick, J. M. Seddon, and G. F. Vancott. 1974. "The Significance of Perineal Pathogens in Women." Journal of Urology 112:808.

Chertok, L., O. Bourgiugnon, F. Guillon, and P. Aboulker. 1977. "Urethral Syndrome in the Female: The Expression of Fantasies about the Urogential Area." Psychosomatic Medicine 39:1.

Cox, C. E. 1966. "The Urethra and Its Relationship to Urinary Tract Infection: The Flora of the Normal Female Urethra." Southern Medical Journal 59:621.

Eisenstaedt, J. S. 1951. "Allergy and Drug Hypersensitivity of the Urinary Tract." Journal of Urology 65:154.

Evans, A. T. 1971. "Etiology of Urethral Syndrome: Preliminary Report." Journal of Urology 105:245.

Farrar, D. J., J. L. Osborne, T. P. Stephenson, G. G. Whiteside, J. Berry, E. Milroy, and T. R. Turner-Warwick. 1976. "A Urodynamic View of Bladder Outflow Obstruction in the Female: Factors Influencing the Results of Treatment." British Journal of Urology 47:815.

Hafner, R. J., S. L. Stanton, and J. Guy. 1977. "A Psychiatric Study of Women with Urgency and Urge Incontinence." British Journal of Urology 49:211.

Hojsgaard, A. 1976. "The Urethral Pressure Profile in Female Patients with Meatal Stenosis." Scandinavian Journal of Urology and Nephrology 10:97.

Horesh, A. 1976. "Allergy and Recurrent Urinary Tract Infections in Childhood." Annals of Allergy 36:16.

Kean, B. H., and W. H. Wolinska. 1956. "Urethral Trichomoniasis: A Cytologic Study." American Journal of Clinical Pathology 26:1142.

Leiter, E. 1973. "Management of Recurrent Cystourethritis in Women." Urology 1:111.

Lipsky, H. 1977. "Urodynamic Assessment of Women with Urethral Syndrome." European Urology 3:202.

Moore, T. 1960. "The Female Prostate: Bladder Neck Obstruction in Women." Lancet 1:1305.

O'Grady, F. W., B. Richards, M. A. McSherry, S. M. O'Farrell, and W. R. Cattell. 1970. "Introital Enterobacteria, Urinary Infection, and the Urethral Syndrome." Lancet 2:1208.

Raz, S., and R. B. Smith. 1976. "External Sphincter Spasticity Syndrome in Female Patients." Journal of Urology 115:443.

Rees, D. L. P., and N. Farhoumand. 1977. "Psychiatric Aspects of Recurrent Cystitis in Women." British Journal of Urology 49:651.

Reiser, C. 1968. "A New Method of Treatment of Inflammatory Lesions of the Female Urethra." Journal of the American Medical Association 204:378.

Richardson, F. H. 1969. "External Urethroplasty in Women: Technique and Clinical Evaluation." Journal of Urology 101: 719.

Roberts, M., and P. Smith. 1968. "Non-malignant Obstruction in the Female Urethra." British Journal of Urology 40:694.

Smith, P. 1972. "Age Changes in the Female Urethra." British Journal of Urology 44:667.

Straub, L. R., H. S. Ripley, and S. Wolf. 1949. "Disturbance of Bladder Function Associated with Emotional States." Journal of the American Medical Association 141:1139.

Tait, A., E. Rees, and R. M. Jameson. 1978. "Urethral Syndrome Associated with Chlamydial Infection of the Urethra and Cervix." British Journal of Urology 50:425.

Tanagho, E., and E. Miller. 1973. "Functional Considerations of Urethral Sphincter Dynamics." Journal of Urology 109:273.

Tanagho, E., E. Miller, R. P. Lyon, and R. Fisher. 1971. "Spastic Striated External Sphincter and Urinary Trade Infection in Girls." British Journal of Urology 43:69.

27

Fear of Death during Rape and the Mourning Process That Follows

Ord Matek
and
Susan E. Kerstein

I was afraid he was going to kill me while it was happening. And now that it's over, there are times I wish he had.

A rape victim

Federal Bureau of Investigation (FBI) statistics indicate that rape is the fastest growing violent crime in the United States and the crime most often committed against women. The Law Enforcement Assistance Administration (LEAA) estimates that between 40 and 50 percent of forcible rapes are not reported, and there are indications that unreported rapes may be as high as 90 percent (Hilberman 1976). According to FBI statistics from 1977, 63,000 rapes were reported to the police for a national rate of 29.1 per 100,000 total population, compared with 9.6 per 100,000 in 1970. Reasons for this increase include an overall increase in the crime and more reporting of rape (Rabkin 1979). The Integrated Criminal Apprehension program funded by LEAA estimated that approximately one woman in six will be subjected to an attempted rape in her lifetime and that one in 24 will be the victim of a completed rape (Nelson 1980).

Women of all ages, marital status, income groups, and professions are raped. The rape is often planned and frequently involves someone the victim knows (Gager and Schurr 1976; Hilberman 1976). Most rapes (53.3 percent) occur in transit, while the victim is going from one place to another or waiting for transportation (Sanders 1980); 14 percent occur either in a socializing context or on a date; and between 20 and 56 percent have been reported to take place at the victim's home (Amir 1971; Sanders 1980). Although rape is usually committed by strangers (68.4 percent of the time), a large percentage of reported rapes (approximately 31.5 percent) and, predictably, a significantly higher proportion of unreported rapes are committed by someone the victim knows: an acquaintance, a neighbor, a friend, or a relative (Amir 1971; Rabkin 1979; Sanders 1980).

These statistics and studies present a frightening profile for women in U.S. society. If rape is unplanned, if it can happen at any time of the day or night, in any place including the victim's home, to any woman, and by someone the victim knows, the feelings of power-lessness, anger, and vulnerability that the victim experiences are in-tensified. The resultant short- and long-term trauma of the attack can be conceptualized as a fear of death during the act and a mourning process afterward.

The opening epigraph for this chapter is a well-articulated, but not unusual, description of the emotional impact of the attack and its aftermath. Although few victims, in fact, actually die as a result of the attack, most victims perceive the attack as a life-threatening ex-perience. All victims regard it as acutely stressful, frightening, and humiliating. Typical statements that reflect the fear of being killed during rape include the following: "My life is disrupted, every part of it upset. But I have to be grateful I wasn't killed. I thought he would murder me" (Burgess and Holmstrom 1974b, p. 983). "He said he'd kill me. He hit me, he choked me, he could [have] kill[ed] me" (Burgess and Holmstrom 1976, p. 415). "I did not struggle, because of the knife. All those things you read about or plan to do don't help. . . . I felt I was not going to get out alive" (Burgess and Holmstrom 1980, p. 37).

In addition to the verbal means, fear of death is further ex-pressed through a variety of somatic, cognitive, and psychological responses. Somatic responses include conscious and unconscious screaming, choking, gagging, nausea, involuntary urinating, hyper-ventilating, and loss of consciousness. "I felt faint, trembling and cold. . . . I went limp" (Burgess and Holmstrom 1976, p. 416). "When I realized what he was going to do, I blanked out" (Burgess and Holmstrom 1980, p. 34).

Burgess and Holmstrom studied the coping behavior of 92 adult female rape victims at three points relative to the attack: during the early awareness of the danger, during the attack itself, and after the attack (1980). The circumstances of the attack, the type of force utilized, and the amount of time between the threat of attack and the actual attack seem to affect the specific cognitive, affective, and/or physical responses of the victim. The victim's responses as they re-late to the attack may influence her ability to move more easily through the normal mourning process that follows.

These same researchers stated that despite the sexual acts or other forms of abuse the victim experiences, survival is the coping task during the attack itself. The woman copes psychologically and manages to survive the attack through depersonalization, dissociation,

denial, suppression, and rationalization. "I kept thinking keep cool.
. . . I said to myself, 'You can handle anything; come on, you can
do it'" (Burgess and Holmstrom 1980, p. 36). Said another victim,
"When I realized what he was going to do, I blanked out . . . tried
not to be aware of what was going on" (Burgess and Holmstrom 1980,
p. 34). Another woman said she still could not believe it happened.

The woman who survives the rape sometimes seems to have experienced a temporary death of her psyche: "I pinched myself to see
if I was real." One woman expressed, "I was resigned, I felt nothing,
empty." Another's response was, "I am missing 10 minutes of my
life" (Burgess and Holmstrom 1976, p. 416). The goal of all living
organisms is adaptation and survival. It appears that by temporarily
killing her psyche, so to speak, the woman allows her body to emerge
alive and she survives. If the victim cannot physically fend off her
attacker, she can adapt to an unpleasant and hostile situation by with-
drawing psychologically.

One way to understand the complex phenomenon wherein the
psyche is extinguished for the sake of survival is from the standpoint
of conservation withdrawal, a concept paralleling some behaviors
found in the animal world. The organism perceives no possibility of
surviving in an inhospitable environment, so it literally shuts down
until such a time that the external environment appears more benign
(Schmale and Engel 1975). Hibernation is an adaptation used by some
animals to tide them over in difficult times. It is the most obvious
example paralleling conservation withdrawal. An even more dramatic
example is tonic immobility, which occurs when a hunted animal becomes paralyzed and immobile when confronted by a predator. The
same sense of paralysis is a common response of many rape victims.
The victim often seems temporarily "frozen" and withdrawn from the
environment. "I was expecting friends and opened my door . . . saw
three men . . . I froze . . . paralyzed for a moment . . . something
went through my head . . . shut the door, but they pushed it back
open . . . with the gun" (Burgess and Holmstrom 1980, p. 34). Similar to the animal trapped in confrontation with an enemy in the wild
and finding itself with no control or means of escape, behavior akin
to the death feint is a dramatic form of adaptation.

Martin Seligman's concept of learned helplessness (1975), derived from learning theory, offers another way to conceptualize this
death of the psyche. He maintains that helplessness is a cognitive-
behavioral response to what is perceived as an adverse environment.
Seligman demonstrated in the laboratory that a creature faced with an
overwhelmingly oppressive environment, realizing that there is ab-
solutely nothing it can do to modify the environment, resigns itself to
whatever torture it experiences. This is a physical submission accompanied by psychological withdrawal.

The rape victim's situation is even more complex. There is anticipatory preparation for her learned helplessness. As a part of her socialization process, the woman has been told by friends, relatives, the media, and the general society to submit to a would-be rapist. "My husband said the guy could kill me or the children . . . but sex wouldn't kill me." Another victim recounted, "I remember talking with people about rape and they always said not to resist . . . that a female could be killed, beaten, or mutilated. I didn't want that to happen" (Burgess and Holmstrom 1976, pp. 415-16). Simultaneously, she has heard from other quarters of society echos of the women's movement telling her that she is a competent human being who has control and power over her life and that she can fight off her attackers.

These mixed messages become even more confusing when rape statistics are analyzed and interpreted. Of the victims who used some type of self-protective measure (spraying Mace, screaming, struggling, fighting back), one-third as many suffered completed rapes compared with those who did not resist. However, two-thirds of the victims who tried to defend themselves suffered more serious injuries in addition to rape (McDermott 1979). In effect, a woman who tries to protect herself may escape the rape, but she also increases the probability that she may receive other injuries in addition to the rape or attempted rape. Clearly, there is no easy direction for the woman who receives this mixed message. She could potentially interpret this information as a no-win situation. Such confusion most likely reinforces the possibility of learned helplessness.

The psychological trauma of rape is caused not only by the sexual aspect of the crime but by a combination of other conditions, which include the suddenness and arbitrariness of the crime, the perceived life-threatening situation by the victim, the apparent purpose of violating the victim's physical integrity and/or rendering her helpless, the victim's forced participation in the intimate act, and the sudden requirement on the victim's part to transcend her normal coping strategies. "In addition to being a violation of the victim's physical self, sexual assault violates the victim's basic beliefs and assumptions about the environment (safe, predictable), about other people and relationships (trust, mutual respect) and about herself (competence, self-confidence and self-esteem)" (Abarbanel 1980, p. 143). These factors compound the trauma of the rape attack and the mourning process that follows.

The crisis of rape disrupts the victim's life physically, emotionally, socially, and sexually; in order to readapt to her environment and achieve a sense of emotional equilibrium, she must work through the crisis of the sexual assault. In effect, the working through becomes a mourning process. As with the death of a loved one, the rape victim has lost a part of herself—albeit a psychological part—and essentially the same unconscious process operates. This is further complicated by concomitant mourning on the part of significant others in the victim's life, who may intrude and sometimes interfere with the victim's mourning (Crenshaw 1978; McCartney 1980; Silverman 1978). There is often blaming of or alienation from the victim by significant others as an unconscious expression of their own and separate mourning experiences. Unlike the bereaved widow who elicits sympathy, the victim of rape experiences accusations by relatives and friends that complicate her mourning.

Freud described mourning as a painful, but normal, function of bereaved persons (1917). Bowlby discussed mourning as a psychological process with fairly predictable behavioral sequences that accompany loss (1961). Mourning is a specific reaction to loss, usually death. It is normal and necessary. The positive by-products of mourning are enhanced when there is full room for expression of anger, guilt, privation, abandonment, and release.

Burgess and Holmstrom called the mourning in the aftermath of attack the rape trauma syndrome (1974a). Although the symptoms (and the order in which they occur) of victims may vary based on individual differences, almost all pass through predictable and sequential phases that represent a normal cycle of emotional response to sexual assault. Whereas all researchers agree that the process the rape victim experiences is the same, they describe and label it in different ways (Burgess and Holmstrom 1974b; Rogers 1978; Sutherland and Scherl 1970).

Burgess and Holmstrom identified a two-stage conceptualization of response patterns in rape victims: an acute phase of disorganization followed by a long-term reorganization process (1974c). Sutherland and Scherl described three phases: acute reaction, "outward or pseudo adjustment," and integration and resolution (1970). Rogers came closest to Kubler-Ross's (1969) mourning process and divided rape victims' responses into five stages: initial, denial, symptom formation, anger, and resolution (1978). (As an aside, the stages that victims pass through are not only theoretical formulations, but as Forman pointed out [1980], they are meaningful in that they give direction to psychotherapy with rape victims.)

The intent of this chapter is to provide an elaboration of the normal mourning process, integrating the ideas of aforementioned researchers and clarifying some aspects of the process. Feinstein proposed a conceptualization of the mourning process by examining three dimensions of the psyche: cognitive, affective, and behavioral (1974, 1975).

The mourning process of rape as perceived by the authors of this chapter builds on Feinstein's model. It has four fluid and somewhat interchangeable phases with indistinct transitions from one phase to another, just as Kubler-Ross (1969) described the mourning stages as flowing back and forth rather than operating on a progressive continuum. In each phase, the victim's psyche can be visualized in a cognitive, affective, and behavioral interaction. Usually, but not always, the mourning process begins at the time of the attack and extends through the resolution phase.

This chapter discusses each phase in detail; it also examines the component parts and the interaction between the phases. For purposes of clarity, we present this material as if each stage is discrete and pure. In actuality, there are always mixed features. The feelings, behaviors, and thoughts identified with each stage are the predominant features of that stage, but they may also occur throughout the process of mourning. They vary in manifestation, intensity, and duration depending on the individual woman's strengths and weaknesses, her support network, and her initial reactions to hospital, legal, and counseling personnel after the attack.

PHASE 1: AWARENESS OF LOSS

Thoughts

In the initial awareness of loss phase, it is impossible for the woman to cope with the stress of the attack without being overwhelmed. Whereas cognitively the woman is confronted with the stress of the moment, it seems necessary for many victims to block out the awareness and feelings of the attack. Thoughts that permit the individual to survive are those that diminish the event or its clarity even while it is happening or for some time afterward. Thoughts such as "This is only a dream" or "This can't be me" depersonalize the experience, make it less real, and may allow only a vague awareness of the event.

Feelings

During the first phase, the affective reaction can be of greater or lesser duration and/or of greater or lesser intensity depending on the victim's circumstances. Burgess and Holmstrom (1974c) identified two styles of the initial response to the attack: a controlled response and an extremely expressive response. It is our belief that Burgess and Holmstrom were really describing the range of affective reactions that can be minimal to maximal. In the controlled or minimal response, the victim appears calm, subdued, or contained; in the expressive or maximal style, she presents as agitated, hysterical, fearful, and visibly upset. Thus, on one end of the continuum is

full denial demonstrated by the nonexpressive style; on the other end
is disbelief or minimal denial demonstrated by florid expression.
Whether victims respond emotionally or nonemotionally, they often
do not want to discuss the rape. This itself represents a variant
form of denial.

Behaviors

Prior to coming to the hospital, some victims try to rid themselves of the experience by bathing or douching and others engage in
routine tasks such as cleaning the house or eating a meal. "Performing routine tasks is a way to reaffirm one's sense of self and/or normalcy; it is a way to regain mastery and control" (Abarbanel 1980,
p. 146). These responses are adaptive and protective. By postpone-
ment, victims give themselves time to prepare for the fullness of the
psychological onslaught later.

During the first few weeks following the rape, the victim may
experience the following acute somatic responses whether or not she
sustained physical injury: soreness, aches, bruises, muscle tension,
vaginal discharge and/or infections, itching, and burning sensation
during urination (Burgess and Holmstrom 1974b, p. 981). These circumstances make continued full denial impossible to maintain, thereby
indefinitely prompting additional responses. However, within a few
days to a few weeks of the attack the victim makes attempts to regain
her sense of equilibrium by resuming normal routines and activities
that she engaged in prior to the attack, thereby demonstrating outward adjustment. Forman compared this to the denial stage an individual encounters in the grieving process (1980).

PHASE 2: RECOGNITION OF LOSS

Although the victim may appear to continue with her old life-
style, she does so in mechanical and superficial ways (Forman 1980).
Cognitively, she begins to recognize a sense of loss and a fuller realization of what happened. At some later point in time, she has a
fuller awareness of its impact in her life and of her own vulnerability.

Phases 2 and 3 of our model are cognitively sequential (see
Table 4). The affective dimension is complicated, however. There
are two possible affective reactions to each cognition. Not all victims feel the same way in response to the same cognition. A trauma
for some initially produces obvious outrage, whereas others need to
withdraw and isolate themselves. Table 4 presents two alternate affective tracks for both cognitions (loss and vulnerability) in order to

TABLE 4

Detail of Mourning Process

Response	Phase 1: Awareness of Loss	Phase 2: Recognition of Loss		Phase 3: Recognition of Vulnerability		Phase 4: Recognition of Survival
Cognitive	"This can't be me" "This is only a dream" "I don't believe this happened"	Flashbacks Preoccupations with rapist Avoidance of locale Desire to move/change phone number Avoidance of friends "Ten minutes of life are missing" "Why me?"		Mistrust of men "Life will never be the same" "Don't know whom to trust" "It can happen anywhere"		"I'm OK" "I'm alive" "I survived"
						Return to feelings of functions: Feeling competent Feeling right about oneself Feeling good
Affective	Disbelief to denial: No feelings Shock Numbness	Track 1: Sadness to depression Guilt Shame Low self-esteem Isolation Anxiety Self-blame	Track 2: Anger to rage Unfocused anger	Track 1: Sadness to depression (same as in phase 2)	Track 2: Anger to rage (same as in phase 2)	
Behavioral response	Defensive actions: Showering Refusal to discuss Douching Normal routines Shock reaction	Track 1: Anorexia Vomiting Sleeplessness Anhedonia Sex dysfunction Nightmares	Track 2: Loss of temper Irritability Impatience Restlessness	(same as in phase 2)		Resumption of normal activities at prerape levels Enrollment in courses Joining women's groups

Note: If victim experiences track 1 in phase 2, then she will respond to track 2 in phase 3, and vice versa.

204

reflect the fact that some rape victims get depressed (track 1) and that others respond with anger (track 2) at different phases in the mourning process. But every woman must traverse both of the phases and tracks in order to complete her mourning process. Again, the intensity-of-feeling reactions in each track should be seen as representing a continuum with a range from "sadness to depression" in one instance and "anger to rage" in the other.

Thoughts

Common cognitions of victims in the recognition-of-loss phase include flashbacks, preoccupations with the assailant, and "Why me?" questions concerning the victimization (Abarbanel 1980; Burgess and Holmstrom 1974b).

Feelings

Guilt and shame are likely to be part of the affective responses observed in track 1 (depression). Notman and Nadelson noted that "a striking phenomenon in rape victims is the initial display of fear, anxiety, guilt, and shame—but little direct anger" (1976, p. 410). Indirect expressions of anger are often demonstrated by the woman's irritability and complaints about treatment. The victim's difficulty in expressing anger and rage directly is a combination of (1) her fears that she provoked the attack and (2) cultural restrictions on women expressing aggression. "Her anger may be repressed and experienced as guilt and shame, despite her concomitant feelings of helplessness" (Notman and Nadelson 1976, p. 410).

Guilt, shame, and self-blame are universal responses to the rape attack. During the initial stages of recovery, the victim searches for reasons or explanations for the assault and how she might have handled the situation differently.

> This struggle to discover why the assault occurred may be seen as an adaptive response. It is a psychological working through of the event. It may be a way to undo what happened. It is also an attempt to retain control. If the victim can establish how and why the assault occurred, she can prevent it from happening again. [Abarbanel 1980, p. 148]

The victim's self-blame is also influenced by society's traditional perception of rape and the rape victim. As a member of society, the woman has accepted the myth that rape only happens to women who "ask for it" or who "let it happen." Even though the woman was forced to participate in the attack, the fact that she participated at all reinforces her self-blame, guilt, and shame. Abarbanel stated that the self-blame represents a choice among alternative explanations for why the assault occurred.

> The fact that rape is a random and arbitrary event is per-
> haps a far more disturbing conclusion than the alternative
> of self-blame. The fact that life is uncertain and people
> are vulnerable to chance events means that victimization
> could happen again. [1980, p. 148]

Guilt in the victim is perpetuated by the fact that society focuses on the sexual rather than the violent aspect of the experience. "Since long-standing sexual taboos still persist for many people, even an un-willing participant in a sexual act is accused and depreciated" (Not-man and Nadelson 1976, p. 410). In addition, it is not uncommon for women to have experienced rape fantasies. Such fantasies are usually pleasurable and, it is important to stress, the fantasized rape is non-violent. However, the truly raped woman may feel that the actual rape is a punishment for her fantasized rape (McCombie 1980, p. 150).

Other common complaints during the recognition-of-loss phase are feelings of isolation and alienation. After the attack, the victim is extremely sensitive to subtle rejections in interpersonal relation-ships.

Behaviors

If the woman first experiences a depressive reaction in this phase (track 1), she is likely to present with physical symptoms—as is the case with any clinical depressive syndrome (headaches, low energy level, sleep disturbances, gastrointestinal irritability, stomach pains, nausea, appetite loss, crying spells, agitation, and sex dys-function).

The more common response for a rape victim is to initially be-come depressed and blame herself, thus following track 1 in the recognition-of-loss phase. Some victims may experience anger and rage (track 2) before they become depressed. For those victims who first have a depressive reaction during the recognition-of-loss phase, anger and rage will become apparent in the third phase of the mourn-ing process, recognition of vulnerability. The alternate track oper-ates for those who felt angry earlier in the second phase, recognition of loss. They will now become more fully in touch with their feelings of depression during phase 3, recognition of vulnerability.

PHASE 3: RECOGNITION OF VULNERABILITY

Thoughts

In the recognition-of-vulnerability phase, the rape victim begins to acknowledge that her life has changed. Many women may think about or actually change residences, jobs, and even friends. Most women must reintegrate their thoughts about men and a general trust in people.

Feelings

Because depression (track 1) has been discussed in terms of phase 2, we will now address the feelings of anger to rage (track 2), which are more commonly—but not always—associated with the recognition-of-vulnerability phase. The anger is not always rational and it is not always focused. It may be diffused and discharged onto everyone and everything in the individual's environment or it may be generalized toward all men; it may be expressed at the helping agents (waiting room staff, hospital staff, social workers, police, therapists); it may even be directed at herself in masochistic acts.

Behaviors

Common behaviors associated with this anger are loss of temper, irritability, impatience, restlessness, and general anxiety. Survival carries the person forward, but she does not see the world as before. She recognizes her vulnerability, a cognition that evokes further adaptive troublesome feelings and a change in many of her behaviors.

PHASE 4: RECOGNITION OF SURVIVAL

Thoughts

As the person moves on to the last phase, recognition of survival, she finally realizes (cognition) that she is a survivor and that life is livable. These thoughts will change some of the woman's affective feelings, which may then return her to more normal functioning. She will never be the same, but she does return to a state of equilibrium. She has begun to more fully integrate the experience into her life and to resolve the trauma of the event. "Resolution is achieved as victims accept the sexual assault as part of their past. The incident itself and circumstances surrounding post-assault behavior should be viewed by victims as a significant life experience, integrated among other experiences" (Forman 1980, p. 310).

While there will be residual scars, issues of trust, concern with the environment, moments of anxiety, and irrational thoughts, they should be manageable if the mourning process has been worked out adequately. Pauline Bart (1981) noted that raped women should no longer be called victims; they are now called survivors in order to emphasize the perceived life-threatening situation of the attack. Such recognition of the woman's survival capacity is reflected in the name we have chosen for the last phase in the mourning process, recognition of survival.

Feelings and Behaviors

During this phase, the woman will regain a feeling of competence and control about herself and her environment. She will have resumed normal routines and activities, and perhaps she will get more involved in groups that help other victims of rape.

Table 4 illustrates some of the specific components of the schema described above.

We have proposed a survival model of coping with the act of rape; in many ways it resembles a model of coping with death. The model is conceptualized as a multiphased mourning process that may begin with the attack. Although researchers have described the normal cycle of response to the rape attack differently, there is uniformity in its meaning. The process involves intense thoughts, feelings, and behaviors in an interrelated configuration. If the woman who survives the attack can successfully pass through these phases, the mourning process will be complete and she can integrate the total experience into her life.

REFERENCES

Abarbanel, G. 1980. "The Roles of the Clinical Social Worker: Hospital Based Management." In Rape and Sexual Assault: Management and Intervention, edited by C. G. Warner, pp. 141-65. Maryland: Aspen Systems.

Amir, M. 1971. Patterns of Forcible Rape. Chicago: University of Chicago Press.

Bart, P. B. 1981. "A Study of Women Who Both Were Raped and Avoided Rape." Journal of Social Issues 37(4): 123–37.

Bowlby, J. 1961. "Processes of Mourning." International Journal of Psychoanalysis 42:317–40.

Burgess, A. W., and L. L. Holmstrom. 1980. "Rape Typology and the Coping Behavior of Rape Victims." In The Rape Crisis Intervention Handbook: A Guide for Victim Care, edited by S. L. McCombie, pp. 27–40. New York: Plenum Press.

_____. 1976. "Coping Behavior of the Rape Victim." American Journal of Psychiatry 133:413–17.

_____. 1974a. "Crisis and Counseling Requests of Rape Victims." Nursing Research 23(3): 196–202.

_____. 1974b. "Rape Trauma Syndrome." American Journal of Psychiatry 131:981–86.

_____. 1974c. Rape: Victims of Crisis. Bowie, Md.: Robert J. Brady.

Crenshaw, T. 1978. "Counseling of Family and Friends." In Rape: Helping the Victim, edited by S. Halpern, D. J. Hicks, and T. L. Crenshaw, pp. 51–60. Oradell, N.J.: Medical Economics.

Feinstein, S. 1975. "Adolescent Depression." In Depression and Human Existence, edited by E. J. Anthony and T. Benedek, pp. 317–36. Boston: Little, Brown.

_____. 1974. "The Effect of Disability on the Adolescent Process." Israel Rehabilitation Annual 11: 37–43.

Forman, B. 1980. "Psychotherapy with Rape Victims." Psychotherapy: Theory, Research and Practice 17(3): 304–11.

Freud, S. 1917. "Mourning and Melancholia." In Standard Edition, vol. 14. London: Hogarth Press.

Gager, N., and C. Schurr. 1976. Sexual Assault: Confronting Rape in America. New York: Grosset & Dunlap.

Hilberman, E. 1976. The Rape Victim. New York: Basic Books.

Kubler-Ross, E. 1969. On Death and Dying. New York: Macmillan.

McCartney, C. F. 1980. "Counseling the Husband and Wife after the Woman Has Been Raped." Medical Aspects of Human Sexuality, May, pp. 121-22.

McCombie, S. L., ed. 1980. The Rape Crisis Intervention Handbook: A Guide for Victim Care. New York: Plenum Press.

McDermott, M. J. 1979. Rape Victimization in 26 American Cities. Albany, N.Y.: U.S. Department of Justice, Criminal Justice Research Center.

Nelson, C. 1980. "Victims of Rape: Who Are They?" In Rape and Sexual Assault: Management and Intervention, edited by C. G. Warner, pp. 9-26. Germantown, Md.: Aspen Systems.

Notman, M. T., and C. C. Nadelson. 1976. "The Rape Victim: Psychodynamic Considerations." American Journal of Psychiatry, April, pp. 408-12.

Rabkin, J. G. 1979. "The Epidemiology of Forcible Rape." American Journal of Orthopsychiatry 49(4): 634-47.

Rogers, P. C. 1978. Rape Counseling Manual. Atlanta: Rape Crisis Center, Grady Memorial Hospital.

Sanders, W. B. 1980. Rape and Women's Identity. Beverly Hills, Calif.: Sage.

Schmale, A. H., and G. L. Engel. 1975. "The Role of Conservation Withdrawal in Depressive Reactions." In Depression and Human Existence, edited by E. J. Anthony and T. Benedek, pp. 183-98. Boston: Little, Brown.

Seligman, M. E. P. 1975. Helplessness: On Depression, Development, and Death. San Francisco: W. H. Freeman.

Silverman, D. C. 1978. "Sharing the Crisis of Rape: Counseling the Mates and Families of Victims." American Journal of Orthopsychiatry 48(1): 166-73.

Sutherland, S., and D. J. Scherl. 1970. "Patterns of Response among Victims of Rape." American Journal of Orthopsychiatry 40: 503-11.

Index

Abarbanel, G. , 205-6
abortion, 5, 76-77, 79, 98, 127,
  162; elective, 98-106; legalization of, 99, 100; research on,
  100-5; selective, 105; services
  for, 99-100, 104; spontaneous,
  63-64, 156 (see also miscarriage); and teenagers, 104
achievement motivation, 11-13, 24
adaptation (see adjustment)
adenocarcinoma, 156, 185
adjustment, 199; to cancer, 176-
  87; parental, and perinatal grief,
  76-79; premorbid, 44
adolescents, 4, 26
age: and adaptation to cancer,
  186; and rape, 197; and social
  support, 179-83; and urethral
  syndrome, 190
aging, 31, 35; and differences
  between sexes, 31-32; and loss,
  30-35; social nature of, 23
American Cancer Society, 134,
  135
amniocentesis, 5
anger, 121, 152, 162-63; bereaved
  child's, 44; at death of spouse,
  39, 40, 173; and DES exposure,
  157; and ectopic pregnancy, 94;
  and elective abortion, 102, 103;
  and gynecologic cancer, 102,
  166, 167-68; toward men, 120;
  in mid-life, 25; following miscarriage, 63; mother's, at stillbirth, 68, 72, 82; and neonatal
  death, 108, 109, 110, 111, 112,
  114; of nursing staff, 89; and
  ovarian cancer, 138, 167; toward psychoanalyst, 120, 121;
  and rape, 198, 201, 205, 206,

207; and selective abortion,
  105; widows', 41, 44, 45
anovulation, 117, 156
anticipatory grief, 152
anticipatory loss, 90, 91
anxiety, 7, 118, 151, 153, 162,
  169; and cancer, 171, 174-75;
  following elective abortion, 102,
  105, 106; following miscarriage,
  74-75, 95; following neonatal
  death, 112, 114; prebirth, 109;
  following rape, 205, 208; following selective abortion, 105;
  and urethral syndrome, 193
attachment, 58, 109

bacterial cystitis, 190, 191
Bart, P. , 208
Beckman, L. J. , 15
bedside manner, 130
Benedek, T. , 116
bereavement, 47, 78, 147, 201;
  anticipatory, 128; and children,
  43-44, 113; correlates of, 76;
  definition of, 39; following elective abortion, 103, 106; and
  perinatal loss, 78 (see also
  perinatal bereavement team);
  process of, 39-40; following
  selective abortion, 105
bereavement care, 147
bereavement file, 84
bereavement groups, 39-40, 41,
  42
bereavement therapy, 37, 41-42,
  47
Berkman, L. F. , and S. L.
  Syme, 175
Berkove, G. F. , 13
biopsy, 142, 149, 181, 185

List of Editors and Contributors

EDITORS

WILLIAM F. FINN, M.D., Associate Professor of Clinical Obstetrics and Gynecology, New York Hospital-Cornell Medical School, New York, New York; Honorary Obstetrician and Gynecologist, North Shore University Hospital, Manhasset, New York

MARGOT TALLMER, Ph.D., Professor, Brookdale Center on Aging, Hunter College of the City University of New York, New York.

IRENE B. SEELAND, M.D., Assistant Clinical Professor of Psychiatry, Department of Psychiatry, College of Physicians and Surgeons, Columbia University, New York, New York

AUSTIN H. KUTSCHER, D.D.S, Professor of Dentistry (in Psychiatry), Department of Psychiatry, College of Physicians and Surgeons, Columbia University, New York, New York; President, The Foundation of Thanatology

ELIZABETH J. CLARK, Ph.D., A.C.S.W., Assistant Professor, Department of Health Professions, Montclair State College, Upper Montclair, New Jersey

CONTRIBUTORS

MARION ADLER, Counselor, Brooklyn, New York

KATHLEEN LEASK CAPITULO, R.N., M.S., Clinical Nurse Specialist, Department of Obstetrics and Gynecology, Booth Memorial Hospital, Flushing, New York

DENIS C. CARLTON, M.S.W., A.C.S.W., The Don Monti Division of Oncology, Department of Medicine, North Shore University Hospital, Manhasset, New York; Department of Medicine, Cornell Medical School, New York, New York

DIANE EATON, C.S.W., Cancer Care, Inc., New York, New York

SELWYN Z. FREED, M.D., Professor and Chairman, Department of Urology, Albert Einstein College of Medicine, Bronx, New York

MAHLON S. HALE, M.D., Associate Professor, Department of Psychiatry, University of Connecticut Health Center, Farmington, Connecticut

JACQUELINE ROSE HOTT, Ph.D., Professor and Codirector, Project for Research in Nursing, Adelphi University School of Nursing, Garden City, New York; Director, Sex Therapy, Family Service Association, Hempstead, New York

SUSAN HUNSDON, A.C.S.W., Department of Social Work Service, The Mount Sinai Hospital and Medical Center, New York, New York

LILA J. KALINICH, M.D., Assistant Clinical Professor of Psychiatry, Department of Psychiatry, College of Physicians and Surgeons, Columbia University, New York, New York

THOMAS D. KERENYI, M.D., Department of Obstetrics and Gynecology, Mount Sinai Hospital and Medical Center, New York, New York

SUSAN E. KERSTEIN, Jane Adams College of Social Work, University of Illinois at Chicago, Chicago, Illinois

LILLIAN G. KUTSCHER, Publications Editor, The Foundation of Thanatology, New York, New York

PHYLLIS C. LEPPERT, M.D., Assistant Professor of Obstetrics and Gynecology, College of Physicians and Surgeons, Columbia University, New York, New York

SUSAN F. LESLIE, New York, New York

GLADYS B. LIPKIN, R.N.C., M.S., F.A.A.N., A.N.A., Certified in Psychiatry/Mental Illness and Obstetrical Nursing, Bayside, New York

NECHAMA LISS-LEVINSON, Ph.D., Psychologist, Great Neck, New York

BARBRA ZUCK LOCKER, M.S., Psychotherapist, Center for Marital and Family Therapy, New York, New York

BRENDA LUKEMAN, Ph.D., Clinical Psychologist, Great Neck, New York

ANTHONY J. MAFFIA, M.S.W., C.S.W., Department of Obstetrics and Gynecology, Booth Memorial Hospital, Flushing, New York

NATHAN MANDELMAN, M.D., Department of Obstetrics and Gynecology, Mount Sinai, Hospital and Medical Center, New York, New York

ORD MATEK, M.A., A.C.S.W., Associate Professor, Jane Adams College of Social Work, University of Illinois at Chicago, Chicago, Illinois

MURIEL G. MORRIS, M.D., Lecturer in Psychiatry, College of Physicians and Surgeons, Columbia University; Columbia University Psychoanalytic Center, New York, New York

JOHN C. MORRISON, M.D., Division of Newborn Medicine, Department of Pediatrics; Division of Maternal-Fetal Medicine, Department of Obstetrics and Gynecology, University of Mississippi Medical Center, Jackson, Mississippi

SUE M. PALMER, M.D., Division of Newborn Medicine, Department of Pediatrics; Division of Maternal-Fetal Medicine, Department of Obstetrics and Gynecology, University of Mississippi Medical Center, Jackson, Mississippi

YVONNE M. PARNES, R.N.C., Nurse Practitioner, Community Health Program of Queens-Nassau, Inc., New Hyde Park, New York

DAVID L. ROSENFELD, M.D., Assistant Professor of Obstetrics and Gynecology, Cornell University Medical Center, New York, New York; Department of Human Reproduction, North Shore University Hospital, Manhasset, New York

JONATHAN SCHER, M.D., Department of Obstetrics and Gynecology, Mount Sinai Hospital and Medical Center, New York, New York

ARLENE SCIORTINO, R.N., The Don Monti Division of Oncology, Department of Medicine, North Shore University Hospital, Manhasset, New York; Department of Medicine, Cornell Medical School, New York, New York

EGILDE SERAVALLI, Ph.D., Department of Anesthesiology, Beth Israel Hospital and Medical Center, New York, New York

DAVID H. SHERMAN, M.D., F.A.C.O.G., Assistant Clinical Professor of Obstetrics and Gynecology, The Mount Sinai School of Medicine, New York, New York

BRENDA C. SUMRALL, A.C.S.W., Division of Newborn Medicine, Department of Pediatrics; Division of Maternal-Fetal Medicine, Department of Obstetrics and Gynecology, University of Mississippi Medical Center, Jackson, Mississippi

VINCENT VINCIGUERRA, M.D., The Don Monti Division of Oncology, Department of Medicine, North Shore University Hospital, Manhasset, New York; Associate Professor of Clinical Medicine, New York Hospital-Cornell Medical School, New York, New York

MARCELLA BAKUR WEINER, Ed.D., Adjunct Professor, Long Island University; Psychotherapist, Brooklyn, New York

CONSTANCE WEISKOPF, R.N., Psychiatric Consultation Service Liaison, Department of Psychiatry, University of Connecticut Health Center, Farmington, Connecticut